THE ANAESTHESIA VIVA

VOLUME 1

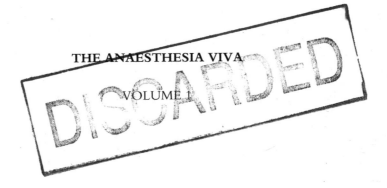

THE ANAESTHESIA VIVA

VOLUME 1

Physiology, Pharmacology & Statistics

John Urquhart
&
Mark Blunt

With contributions from Mark Dixon

⅃GℳℳꙆ

© 1996
Greenwich Medical Media
507 The Lincn Hall
162-168 Regent Street
London
W1R 5TB

ISBN 1 900 15100 6

First Published 1996

A catalogue record for this book is available from the British Library

Distributed worldwide by
Oxford University Press

Typeset and Designed by
Derek Virtue, DataNet

Printed in Great Britain by
Derry Print Limited

PREFACE

The Royal College of Anaesthetists has revised its schedule for the FRCA examination from three parts to two, which , from 1996, will be called the Primary and the Final FRCA. The "new" primary examination syllabus includes basic anaesthesia and resuscitation, an OSCE, and has ten pages devoted to Anatomy, Physiology, Physics, Clinical Measurement and Basic Statistics. This formidable syllabus and the list of basic science subjects is in itself a daunting proposition for many prospective trainee anaesthetists. This book of Questions and Answers for the new primary FRCA examination provides an impressive catalogue of well illustrated material for candidates contemplating the physiology and pharmacology parts of the examination. The book is equally relevant in the oral as well as the written part of this examination and is based on an extensive experience of the authors in teaching candidates for the basic science parts of previous FRCA examinations. The authors have the advantage that they are clinicians teaching basic sciences and they have chosen topics from their experience of questions asked in the examination as well as topics which have particular clinician relevance. Many candidates for this part of the examination as well as their consultant teachers may see little clinical relevance of many parts of the basic science section of the syllabus for the new primary.

The present book provides an excellent preview of the range of knowledge presently expected by candidates for the new primary. It should not be regarded as a substitute for traditional text books but it is an important supplement to such reading. It is certainly a very useful way to revise and particularly valuable for practising the viva voce part of the examination. Many candidates fail not because of lack of knowledge of the facts but because of lack of practice in oral question and answer sessions. Many senior colleagues would like to help their trainees with the oral part of the examination but they have forgotten the scope and detail of the basic science part of the examination and this book again provides a treasure chest of questions for the mock examiner. I look forward to further editions which will include other parts of the new primary syllabus.

Professor Gareth Jones,
Cambridge, 1996

CONTENTS

3. QUESTIONS IN
RESPIRATORY PHYSIOLOGY

6. QUESTIONS ON
   RENAL PHYSIOLOGY

7. QUESTIONS IN METABOLIC
   PHYSIOLOGY AND BIOCHEMISTRY

8. QUESTIONS ON
   ANAESTHETIC DRUGS

9. QUESTIONS ON
PHARMACOKINETICS AND PHARMACODYNAMICS

10. QUESTIONS ON CARDIOVASCULAR PHARMACOLOGY

11. QUESTIONS ON MOLECULAR PHARMACOLOGY

12. QUESTIONS ON THE PHARMACOLOGY OF THE NEUROMUSCULAR JUNCTION

13. QUESTIONS ON
NON-ANAESTHETIC DRUGS

14. QUESTIONS ON STATISTICS

APPENDIX 1:

APPENDIX 2:

APPENDIX 3:

INDEX

VOLUME 1

THE ANAESTHESIA VIVA
(PHYSIOLOGY, PHARMACOLOGY & STATISTICS)

This book is the result of teaching candidates for the second part of the old series of examinations for the Fellowship of the Royal College of Anaesthetists. The viva examination for many people remains a daunting prospect, we hope that this book will help to reduce the anxiety that all candidates feel as they walk into the examination hall.

The passing of any examination is probably 70% knowledge, 20% technique and 10% luck. There are some excellent pharmacology and physiology textbooks available, but they do not present information in a form that answers a question, and this is what this book sets out to provide.

Some points bear emphasis. Look smart, speak clearly to the examiner, and do not mumble. Make eye contact, and appear confident. Saying "may I have a piece of paper" in response to a question requiring a graph or diagram impresses. Make a remark by way of an overview, while mentally accumulating your answer. Many of the answers in the text do this, and such remarks and other vital facts, are denoted thus:

➡ **Apart from buying thinking time, an overview demonstrates to an examiner that you know what you are talking about.**

For example, in response to the question, "What is a buffer?" it is impossible to begin to score points by stating that the pKa of the bicarbonate buffer is 6.1; a buffer consists of a weak acid with the conjugate base, and such a definition puts you onto safe ground. Most questions will begin simply; you might be asked "what induction agent do you use?" This is an invitation to discuss the one you know most about. The point about such questions is that they are a means of starting to explore your knowledge; you are expected to be able to talk about an induction agent, but what they want to talk about is how the induction agent works, about receptor theory, about the basis of anaesthesia perhaps.

The questions are arranged by system. They are, for the most part, not opening questions like the one above, but rather, they follow the line the discussion would take. However, for simplicity, they are presented as questions - but think of them as supplementary to a starter question. Diagrams are offered and every attempt has been made to make them as simple as possible so that a candidate might be able to reproduce them in the exam. However, there are some more complicated diagrams that are of a complexity not required for the exam but that help the explanations.

Finally, this is not a definitive text for the Primary exam. It is a collection of answers to some of the questions that have been asked, and it is our hope that it should provide a few guidelines to the way to go about the viva exam.

1 QUESTIONS IN THE PHYSIOLOGY OF THE CENTRAL NERVOUS SYSTEM

1. DEFINE THE FOLLOWING:

1. Anaesthesia.
2. Pain.
3. Analgesia.
4. Sedation.

- **Anaesthesia** is the absence of cerebral response to a painful stimulus. (Note that a patient who is 'aware' is therefore not under anaesthesia, and that anaesthesia may be produced by inhibition of neuronal transmission at a number of different levels).
- **Pain** is an unpleasant sensory and emotional experience associated with actual or potential tissue damage, or described in terms of such damage.
- **Analgesia** is the absence of pain on noxious stimulation.
- **Sedation** is a reduction of the level of consciousness, usually by pharmacological means, such that the patient is still able to respond to verbal command.

....

2. WHAT IS A SENSORY MODALITY?

➡ **A sensory modality is a type of sensation, and may have sub-modalities; for example touch has the submodalities of light touch, pressure and vibration.**

A reflex is an automatic, appropriate, stereotyped response. It is usually graded and under descending inhibitory control.

A sensory unit is a single axon leading back to the dorsal horn from a number of receptors. It serves a receptive field. The more densely innervated an area of skin, the smaller the receptive field and the finer the sensation.

....

3. CAN YOU DISCUSS SMOOTH MUSCLE ACTION POTENTIAL AND INNERVATION?

➡ **The Action Potential may be one of two types: Spikes and plateaux.**

1. Spikes are seen in tubular structures such as the gut and the ureters. They are superimposed on slow waves which have a latency of up to 10 seconds.

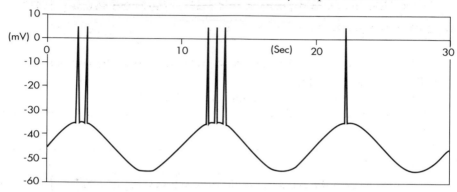

2. Plateaux are seen in the heart (the cardiac action potential) and the uterus.

Differences in the action potential between smooth muscle and skeletal muscle:

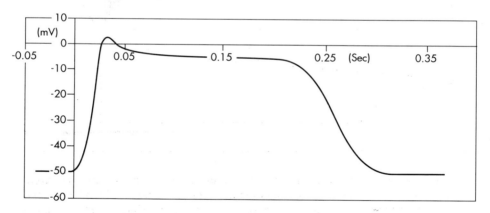

a. There is an oscillating resting potential in smooth muscle.

b. Resting potential in smooth muscle is –60mV (-85 mV in skeletal muscle).

c. Prolonged relaxation is a feature of smooth muscle.

d. Tension may be maintained for longer in smooth muscle than skeletal muscle.

e. Smooth muscle uses less ATP.

Innervation: There are two patterns in smooth muscle

- Contact type: This is analogous to skeletal muscle.
- Diffuse type: Terminal nerve fibres wind their way through smooth muscle mass or into fibrous tissue around it, but never penetrate the muscle tissue.

● ●

4. CAN YOU DESCRIBE THE CONTROL OF CEREBRAL BLOOD FLOW?

➡ **The key to this subject is the understanding of intracranial pressure (ICP). This is the pressure within the vault of the skull, and is normally 10-15 cmH$_2$O in the prone or supine positions. Anaesthesia for intra cranial operations requires conditions which maintain perfusion of the brain. This in turn is dependant on Cerebral Perfusion Pressure (CPP).**

➡ **CPP = MAP - (ICP + CVP)**

(where MAP = Mean Arterial Pressure, which is Diastolic + 0.3 Pulse Pressure)

- The brain weighs 1500 grams
- Normal cerebral blood flow is 750ml min^{-1} (50ml/100g tissue)
- Oxygen consumption (VO$_2$) for cerebral tissue is 50ml min^{-1} (3.5ml/100g tissue)

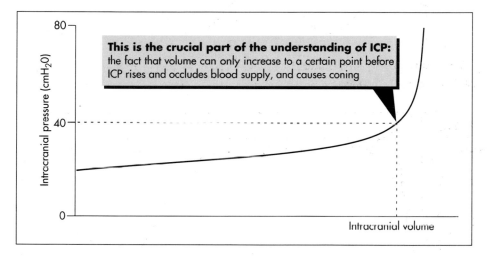

This is the crucial part of the understanding of ICP: the fact that volume can only increase to a certain point before ICP rises and occludes blood supply, and causes coning

Autoregulation is the ability of the brain (or of any tissue) to control its own blood supply - Cerebral Blood Flow, CBF, autoregulates within certain limits. The cerebral arterioles constrict as the cerebral arterial pressure rises, protecting against too high a pressure, and dilate as the pressure diminishes, allowing more blood to perfuse the brain. This operates between MAP of 60-130 mmHg, which is why the MAP is the most useful reading (as well as the most accurate) on the Dinamap. Autoregulation, and the protection it provides, is abolished by hypoxia, hypercapnia and trauma, and also to a degree by volatile anaesthetic agents. It may sometimes be restored by hyperventilation.

. . . .

5. WHAT IS THE MECHANISM OF THE KNEE JERK?

➡ **This is about the muscle spindle → Dorsal horn → motor nerve reflex arc.**

The intrafusal fibre is the receptor component of the reflex. It is embedded within the skeletal muscle fibre. It is innervated by Aγ fibres which cause tightening of the fibre. The central sensory part is innervated by Aα fibres, which are fast, primary fibres to the cord, and by slower, β fibres to the cortex.

Static response:

Receptor portion is stretched, a signal is transmitted for a prolonged period of time via the slow, β type fibres from the receptor portion.

Dynamic response:

This is the response to rate of change; a signal is transmitted only during the change in length, via fast, primary, Aα fibres.

If extrafusal fibre length becomes greater than intrafusal fibre length:

→ Receptor is stretched to accommodate this change in length.

→ Increased afferent signal

If intrafusal fibre length becomes greater than extrafusal fibre length:

→ The receptor is slack

→ Decreased afferent signal

Which is opposed by: The Golgi tendon organ

- These lie in the tendon of a muscle at the tendon-muscle junction.
- The Golgi tendon organ responds to tension whereas the muscle spindle responds to length.
- The Golgi tendon organ sends inhibitory signals whereas the muscle spindle sends excitatory signals.
- It probably sets a protective function on the muscles preventing damage.

....

6. WHAT CAUSES THE MAINTENANCE OF MUSCLE TONE?

➡ **This is achieved by summation, which is the adding together of individual muscle twitches to make strong and concerted movements.**

There are two types of summation:

1. Multiple motor unit summation, which involves increasing the number of motor units contracting simultaneously.
2. Increasing the rapidity of contraction, which is known as wave summation.

....

7. WHAT IS THE DIFFERENCE BETWEEN THE ACTION POTENTIALS OF NERVE AND MUSCLE?

1. The resting potential is about –85mV in muscles and in the large nucleated fibres that supply them.
2. The duration in muscle is 5ms, which is five times as long as that in the nerve.
3. The velocity of transmission in muscle is $5ms^{-1}$, this is 1/18 the velocity of nerve transmission.

The action potential in muscle travels longitudinally and then down the T-tubules which are extracellular; however they become adjacent to the cisternae at the ends of the sarcoplasmic reticulum. The cisternae release Ca^{++} ions which interact with the troponin and cause contraction. A calcium pump then returns the Ca^{++} to the sarcoplasmic reticulum.

....

8. DISCUSS THE PERIPHERAL PAIN PATHWAYS.

You would not be asked this question in this form, but an overview may be useful.

Nociceptors - if you believe in them (cornea has none)

Aδ - fast, myelinated afferent nerve fibres (40 m/sec)
C - slow, unmyelinated afferent nerve fibres (2 m/sec)

In the substantia gelatinosa C fibres have projections which terminate and participate in the gate theory, which is that substansia gelatinosa cells have an inhibitory effect on 'target' cells which are the cells which project onto the thalamus. Target cells are stimulated by both C and Aδ fibres. SG cells are stimulated by Aβ fibres and so Aβ stimulation can inhibit pain perception by 'closing' the gate hence -

• The effects of "rubbing pain better"

• TENS (**t**ranscutaneous **e**lectrical **n**erve **s**timulation)

This is **NOT** opposed by naxolone, since no opiate receptors are involved

Thereafter - pathways cross at same levels ➡ lateral spinothalmic tract ➡ thalamus ➡ cortex

Aδ fibres project onto neurones which in turn project directly to higher centres.

....

9. WHAT ARE THE FUNCTIONS OF THE VAGUS NERVE?

➡ **These are motor, sensory and secretomotor.**

Motor, to:
- Larynx.
- Bronchial muscles.
- Alimentary tract (as far as the splenic flexure).
- Myocardium.

Sensory, to:
- Dura.
- External auditory meatus.
- Respiratory tract.
- Alimentary tract (to ascending colon).
- Myocardium.
- Epiglottis.

Secretomotor:
- Bronchial mucus production.
- Alimentary tract and adnexa.

....

10. WHAT ARE THE FUNCTIONS OF THE EXTRAPYRAMIDAL SYSTEM?

➡ **The extrapyramidal system:**
- **Regulates muscle tone.**
- **Governs stereotyped movements.**

It consists of:

Subcortical nuclei
Caudate nucleus
Globus pallidus ⎫ These are the basal ganglia.
Putamen
Brain stem nuclei

Rubrobulbar tract ⎫ These tracts accompany upper motor neurones to
Reticulospinal tract ⎭ influence lower motor neurone pathways.

Tectospinal tract ⎫ These adjust for eye and ear movement.
Vestibulospinal tract ⎭

It is so called because it is ***not*** part of that system which forms the pyramid of the medulla

....

11. WHAT IS THE BLOOD - BRAIN BARRIER?

➡ **The blood-brain barrier (BBB) resides in the endothelial cells lining the cerebral capillaries; the endothelium is sealed by tight junctions.**

Unlike a desmosome, the tight junction is circumferential. Thus, all transport must be transcellular.

The BBB is deficient in the region of the chemoreceptor trigger zone (CTZ).

- Lipid- soluble drugs cross the BBB easily.
- The transport of amino acids and glucose is carrier mediated.

••••••••••••••••••••••••••••••

12. WHAT IS THE EFFECT ON MUSCLE OF HYPERVENTILATION?

➡ **This is about tetany.**

Primary effect:

- Rise in PaO_2 (but not necessarily a rise in SpO_2) because of reduced P_ACO_2.
- Fall in $PaCO_2$ which leads to vasoconstriction and a rise in systemic vascular resistance, which will include cerebral vasoconstriction and result in loss of consciousness.

Secondary effect: Alkalosis, due to reduction in $PaCO_2$.

Calcium is in the plasma in free ionised, and protein-bound forms; of these it is the ionised form which is physiologically active.

- As pH falls (the environment becomes more acidic) so [Ca^{++}] rises as it is displaced from protein binding.
- As pH rises (i.e. less free H$^+$) so [Ca^{++}] falls.

The low Ca^{++} causes excitation in the muscle cell leading to clonus and eventually to uncontrolled muscular contraction.

The tendency to tetany may be quantified as being proportional to:

$$\frac{[HCO_3^-] \times [HPO_4^-]}{[Ca^{++}] \times [Mg^{++}] \times [H^+]}$$

••••••••••••••••••••••••••••••

13. WHAT IS THE RETICULAR ACTIVATING SYSTEM?

➡ **The reticular activating system (RAS) is a loosely arranged collection of fibres and cells in the Brainstem.**

1. The RAS receives and integrates information from all parts of the central nervous system (CNS).
2. The RAS outputs information to all parts of the CNS.
3. The RAS is responsible for arousal and RAS activity is implicated in the level of consciousness.

Definitions:

Forebrain   = Cerebrum + diencephalon.

Diencephalon = Thalamus + hypothalamus.

Brainstem   = Midbrain + pons + medulla.

There are projections of the RAS to:

- Thalamus.
- Cortex, directly.

There is convergence onto the RAS from:

- Sensory tracts.
- The trigeminal nerve.
- The auditory nerve.
- The olfactory nerve.

•••••••••••••••••••••••••••••••

14. WHAT NERVE FIBRES DO YOU RECOGNISE?

Class	Function	Size (mm diameter)	Velocity (m/sec)
Aα	Somatic motor	12-20	70-120
Aβ	Touch, pressure, proprio'n	5-12	30-70
Aγ	Spindle afferents	3- 6	15-30
Aδ	Sharp pain, Temperature	2- 5	12-30
B	Preganglionic autonomic	<3	3-15
C	Dull pain	0.4-1.2	0.5-2.0

Local anaesthetics block small fibres before large ones; pressure affects large fibres before small ones. This is why a motor palsy with preservation of sensation may be a consequence of pressure trauma.

•••••••••••••••••••••••••••••••

15. DESCRIBE THE NEURONAL PATHWAYS THAT ARE INVOLVED IN THE INITIATION OF A VOLUNTARY MOVEMENT.

➡ **Voluntary movement starts in the *motor cortex* (pre-central gyrus), but the thought behind that movement starts from the *supplementary motor area* or pre-motor area.**

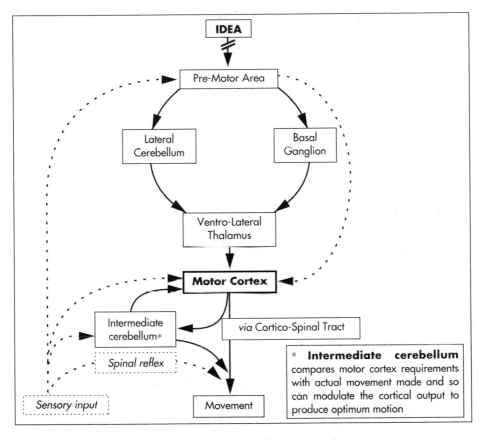

The impulse then descends through the **internal capsule** before decussating into the **cortico-spinal tract** to the anterior horn cell and then to the α– **motor neurone**.

Within the corticospinal tract there is branching to help produce multiple innervation and so produce a controlled movement.

•••••••••••••••••••••••••••••

16. EXPLAIN WHY A GUARDSMAN DOES NOT FALL OVER.

➡ **This is a question about the maintenance of upright posture, and specifically what reflexes are used to maintain that position.**

1. Spinal Cord reflexes.
   - Stretch receptors exert negative feedback to maintain position (e.g. at the ankle).
   - Cutaneous receptors in feet also exert negative feedback.
   - Joint receptors; negative feedback.
   - Interlimb receptors: These produce a reflex effect in the contralateral limb after movement on one side.

2. Vestibular and Vestibulospinal reflexes; these activate limb muscles to help maintain the head's position in space, and limb movements to help by counter-balancing any movement.

3. Neck reflexes are very strong stretch reflexes.

4. Vestibulo–Ocular reflex; this enables the eyes to move to cancel out head motion, so the retinal picture remains constant whilst head movement occurs.

5. The opticokinetic reflex is a higher function reflex that relates body position to visual movement. So if the guardsman's whole visual field moves backward suddenly (the picture he would get if he were falling forwards) the reflex will move him backwards strongly.

·····························

2 QUESTIONS IN CARDIOVASCULAR PHYSIOLOGY

1. HOW DO YOU MEASURE BLOOD VOLUME?

➡ **A repeatable method of measurement would be a considerable advance in medical science but does not exist.**

One technique uses a known volume of ^{51}Cr-radiolabelled red cells, which are injected into the circulation and allowed to equilibrate. A sample is taken later, and the blood volume may be calculated from:

$$\text{Blood volume in ml} = \frac{\text{Quantity of test substance injected}}{\text{Concentration of test substance observed}}$$

Where the test substance is the labelled red cells.

An alternative technique involves the use of either radio-labelled albumin or Evans blue. Albumin will eventually distribute outside the vascular compartment, but to begin with it will reside in the plasma. The same mathematics is applied, but the measurement obtained is of course a measurement of plasma volume. In order to know the volume of blood, this equation is applied:

$$\text{Blood volume in ml} = \text{plasma volume} \times \frac{100}{100 - \text{haematocrit.}}$$

··

2. WHAT IS NORMAL MYOCARDIAL ENERGY SUBSTRATE?

➡ **Oxygen stored in the myoglobin provides only a modest reserve.**

Less than 1% of energy is derived anaerobically, up to maximum of 100% during hypoxia; however under anoxic conditions the energy liberated is insufficient to cause contractions, but may not cause immediate cell death.

> 35% by carbohydrate
> 5% by ketones   } Basally
> 60% by fats

After glucose loading, the heart can use large quantities of lactate and pyruvate. During starvation, it can use a large proportion of fatty acids.

··

3. WHAT IS THE EFFECT OF SEVERE HAEMORRHAGE ON PULMONARY FUNCTION?

1. Hyperventilation, due to the acidosis which is a consequence of hypovolaemia and regional underperfusion.
2. Hypoxic pulmonary vasoconstriction, which is a paradox in this case, as it causes increased V/Q mismatch and further deterioration in pulmonary function.
3. There is an increase in respiratory dead space.
4. Oxygen hunger, which is a gasping deep respiration, and represents a chemoreceptor response to hypotension.

....

4. WHAT IS THE FICK PRINCIPLE?

➡ **The Fick principle states that the amount of a substance taken up by an organ (or by the whole body) per unit of time is equal to the arterial level of the substance minus the venous level multiplied by the blood flow.**

➡ **It can be employed to calculate blood flow, in the knowledge of the other variables, or to calculate $\dot{V}O_2$, oxygen consumption.**

By taking simultaneous arterial and mixed venous samples it is possible to derive the difference in oxygen content. Mixed venous blood may be taken from the tip of a pulmonary artery (PA) catheter, or from a catheter in the right ventricle. Blood from the PA may contain shunted blood, however, which will lead to inaccuracies.

$$\dot{Q} = \frac{\dot{V}O_2}{(CaO_2 - C\bar{v}O_2)}$$

For CaO_2 and $C\bar{v}O_2$:

$$O_2 \text{ content} = (1.31 \times Hb \times \text{Saturation} /100) + 0.002 \, PO_2$$

The $\dot{V}O_2$ can then be assessed in the light of the cardiac output at that time. Shoemaker *(Intensive Care Med* (1987) **13**:230-243) suggests that the critically ill patient requires a $\dot{V}O_2$ 30% greater than normal (N = 100 - 180 ml/min/m^2). This is contentious however and many regard the Shoemaker criteria as a physiological trial rather than a set of goals.

....

5. WHAT IS MIXED VENOUS OXYGEN SATURATION?

➡️ **Mixed venous oxygen saturation is the percentage of mixed venous blood which is oxygenated, and may be measured photometrically at the tip of a Pulmonary Artery (PA) catheter.**

S$\bar{v}$O$_2$ is decreased with:

1. Anaemia.
2. Low cardiac output.
3. Arterial oxygen desaturation.
4. Increased oxygen consumption.

S$\bar{v}$O$_2$ is increased with:

1. Sepsis with peripheral shunting.
2. Cyanide toxicity.
3. Hypothermia.
4. A wedged PA catheter.

(From TE Oh, *Intensive Care Manual*, 3rd Ed)

....

6. CAN YOU DRAW THE BLOOD COAGULATION PATHWAYS?

➡️ **Primary haemostasis depends solely on platelet function. The coagulation proteins form fibrin which stabilises the platelet clot.**

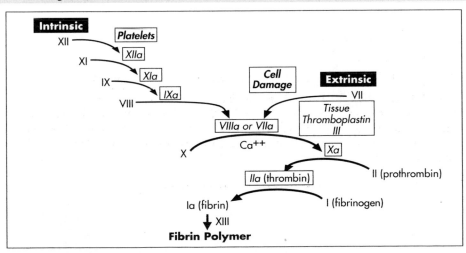

The intrinsic pathway is so-called because all components circulate in plasma (items in white boxes act as catalysts on, or initiators of, the reactions shown).

....

7. WHAT ARE THE CAUSES OF BRADYCARDIA UNDER ANAESTHESIA?

➡ **The most important cause of bradycardia under anaesthesia is hypoxia. It may also be due to surgical, drug-related, metabolic or disease-related causes.**

Surgical:

1. Ophthalmic; traction of extra-ocular muscle
2. Mesenteric traction
3. Anal stretch

} These are vagally-mediated, and seen especially in children

Drugs:

1. Halothane.
2. Neostigmine.
3. Suxamethonium, with special reference to the second dose.
4. Spinal blockade at T1-T4 , which is seen in:
   - Spinal anaesthesia.
   - Spinal injuries.

Metabolic:

1. Hypothyroidism.
2. Hyperkalaemia.

Disease:

1. Ischaemic heart disease.
2. Raised intracranial pressure.

••••••••••••••••••••••••••••••

8. WHAT TESTS OF COAGULATION DO YOU USE?

1. Platelet count: Normal is greater than $150000/mm^3$.
2. Fibrinogen: Normal is greater than 150 mg/100 ml.
3. Platelet function: Bleeding time should be leass than 10 min.
4. Intrinsic pathway: Activated partial thromboplastin time (APTT)   should be less than 38 seconds.
5. Extrinsic pathway: Prothrombin time (PT) should be less than 16 seconds. This may also be given as the International Normalised Ratio (INR) to a control using a standard thromboplastin. The ratio required depends on the condition, e.g. 2 for embolic prophylaxis in atrial fibrillation, 3 for a prosthetic valve.

Individual coagulation factors may be assayed but these are not routine tests. The thromboelastograph is an interesting tool but do not mention it unless you can talk about it with authority.

••••••••••••••••••••••••••••••

9. HOW DO ANTICOAGULANTS AFFECT THESE TESTS OF COAGULATION?

WARFARIN: Prolongs the PT.

This is a vitamin K antagonist, causing false synthesis of γ-carboxyglutamic acid residues at the factors listed below. Note the length of the half-life ($t_{1/2}$) for each factor; this is why the action of warfarin is so long:

- VII: $t_{1/2}$ 2 h;
- X: $t_{1/2}$ 17 h;
- X: $t_{1/2}$ 40 h;
- II: $t_{1/2}$ 60 h.

Dose: 10 mg od, until adequate INR is achieved, then maintenance with ¼ total initial dose. Reversal may be achieved with Vitamin K 10 mg and Fresh Frozen Plasma (FFP) if urgent.

HEPARIN: Prolongs the APTT.

This is an antithrombin III cofactor; 100 u = 1 mg. Initial dose is 5000 u, then 1000 u/hr. Reversal by Protamine 1 mg/100 u heparin.

LOW MOLECULAR WEIGHT HEPARIN: Need factor X assay to monitor effect.

This consists of fractionated heparin, is a once daily dose, and is said to be more effective in orthopaedic practice. It is less reversible with protamine than is conventional heparin.

••••••••••••••••••••••••••••••••

10. WHAT IS THROMBOLYSIS?

➡ **Thrombolysis is the dissolution of a stable clot or thrombus.**

Vascular endothelium produces prostacyclin, which is a platelet inhibitor.

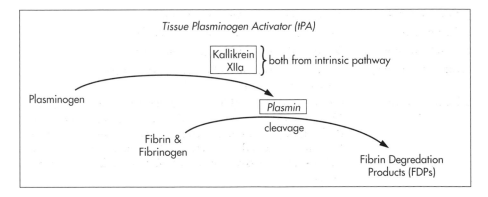

(Items in white boxes act as catalysts on, or initiatiors of, the reactions shown).

••••••••••••••••••••••••••••••••

11. WHAT METHODS ARE THERE FOR THE MEASUREMENT OF CARDIAC OUTPUT?

➡ **This question would then lead into discussion of one method. Be well informed on one – thermodilution is the safest.**

1. Thermodilution. Assume cardiac output from the right ventricle is the same as from the left.

Through the proximal port of a pulmonary artery catheter, inject iced water or saline; at the tip of the catheter is a thermistor.

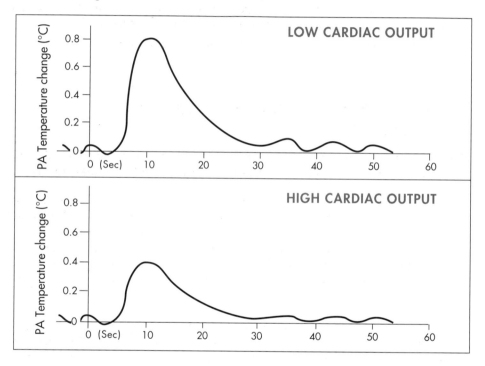

Cardiac output a 1/area under the curve (AUC).

2. Fick: this is cumbersome – Fick is usually used to calculated $\dot{V}O_2$ using CO.

3. Doppler Echo: calculates stroke volume, which is then multiplied by heart rate to give cardiac output. Doppler is very inaccurate.

4. Bioimpedance. Usually regarded as a research tool.

••••••••••••••••••••••••••••••

12. WHAT ARE THE DETERMINANTS OF OXYGEN FLUX?

➡ **Oxygen Flux = Cardiac output x Arterial oxygen content.**

This is not the same as $\dot{V}O_2$.

O_2 content (ml/dl blood)= $(1.31^\star x\ Hb\ x\ Saturation/100) + 0.02\ PO_2$

★ this is the oxygen content of one haemoglobin molcule when fully saturated. The actual figure is quoted variously between 1.31 and 1.39 (ml O_2/g haemoglobin).

0.02 is the solubility coefficient of oxygen in blood at 37°C and is used to show the oxygen carried in solution in both reythrocyes and plasma (ml/dl per kPa).

Often quoted as an index, i.e. per m^2 of Body Surface Area (BSA).

....

13. WHAT CHANGES OCCUR IN RESPONSE TO TRAINING?

➡ **Training results in a predictable pattern of multisystemic changes affecting the cardiovascular, respiratory and musculoskeletal systems.**

1. Maximal O_2 uptake increases. Maximal Breathing Capacity usually exceeds pulmonary ventilation at maximal exercise. The limiting factor is cardiac output and O_2 delivery; however O_2 diffusing capacity also increases.

2. Marathon runners can achieve a maximal Cardiac Output (CO) about 40% greater than untrained people. This occurs by an increase in heart muscle mass and an increase in heart size. End-diastolic volume and stroke volume both increase. This is why at rest the trained person has a lower heart rate than the untrained person.

3. There is an increase in muscle mass due to hypertrophy of individual muscle fibres, more storage of glycogen and proliferation of capillaries. The increased number of capillaries decreases intercapillary distance and allows improved blood supply during exercise. As a consequence O_2 debt only occurs later in exercise.

....

14. WHAT ARE THE FUNCTIONS OF PLATELETS?

➡ **Platelets are formed from bone marrow megakaryocytes.**

1. Platelet plug: collagen contact causes ADP release which causes platelet activation.

2. Platelets are involved in histamine storage and release.

3. Thromboxanes – these cause platelet adhesion (cyclo-oxygenase function; arachidonic acid metabolism.)

4. Platelet – derived growth factor (PDGF) stimulates wound healing and is a mitogen for vascular smooth muscle.

....

15. WHAT DOES A PULMONARY ARTERY FLOTATION CATHETER MEASURE DIRECTLY AND WHAT CAN BE DERIVED?

➡ **It measures temperature and pressure and is directed into the pulmonary artery by the flow of blood.**

After inflation of the balloon, pulmonary capillary wedge pressure (PCWP) can be measured from which left atrial pressure is inferred giving an indication of left ventricular end diastolic volume (LVEDV), which relates to fibre length at the start of systole.

Indirectly, you need central venous pressure (CVP) and systemic arterial pressure. Cardiac output from the right ventricle is measured by thermodilution, being inversely proportional to the area under the curve.

Cardiac index	CI	=	CO/BSA
	SVR	=	(MAP - CVP) /CO x 80
	SVRI	=	(MAP - CVP) /CI x 80
	PVR	=	(MPAP - PCWP) /CO x 80
	PVRI	=	(MPAP - PCWP) /CI x 80
	SI	=	CI/HR
	LVSWI	=	SI x (MAP –PCWP) x 0.0136
	RVSWI	=	SI x (MPAP - CVP) x 0.0136

· ·

16. WHAT IS CONTRACTILITY AND HOW DO WE DETERMINE IT?

➡ **Contractility refers to the inotropic state of the heart independant of end–diastolic volume, heart rate and systemic vascular resistance.**

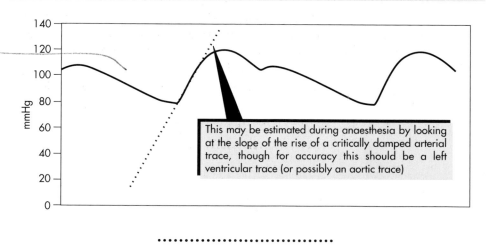

This may be estimated during anaesthesia by looking at the slope of the rise of a critically damped arterial trace, though for accuracy this should be a left ventricular trace (or possibly an aortic trace)

· ·

17. HOW IS BLOOD STORED?

All donated blood starts as 450 ml from the donor, with 60 ml additive, cooled to 4°.
CAPD = citrate, adenine, phosphate, dextrose
SAGM = sodium chloride, adenine, glucose, mannitol
Random blood   64.0%   compatible
ABO XM   99.4%   compatible
ABO + Rh XM 99.8%   compatible
Full XM   99.95% compatible
(XM= Crossmatch)

PRODUCT	VOLUME (ml)	ADDITIVE	HCT	LIFE
Whole blood	450	60 ml CAPD	0.45	21 days
Plasma-reduced blood	350	60 ml CAPD	0.60	21 days
SAGM	200	100 ml SAGM	0.60	45 days
Concentrated red cells	200	minimum	0.80	21 days
Human Albumin	450	pasteurised 60°C		6 months
Fresh Frozen Plasma (contains all factors)	200	stored at -30°C		6 months
Cryoprecipitate (factor VIII especially)	15	stored at -30°C		6 months
Platelets	1 unit whole blood provides 1 unit platelets; 6 units of platelets ↑ platelet count by 30,000			3 days

Stored blood: pH 6.9, K^+ 20 mmol/l, HCO_3 10 mmol/l.
Filters in giving sets: A100 = 180 μm; depth or screen = 20–40 μm.

. . . .

18. WHAT ARE THE FUNCTIONS OF LYMPHATICS?

1. To return interstitial fluid to the circulation as lymph. Lymphatic capillaries do not have tubes flowing into them, unlike blood capillaries. There are one–way valves governing the flow into the cisterna chyli from the lymphatic duct.

2. Lymph nodes are a focus of immune activity.

3. The total generated is 4L lymph/day, which acts to prevent the formation of oedema.

4. Lymphatics are responsible for the absorption of fat from intestine.

. . . .

19. CAN YOU DRAW THE PRESSURE CURVES FOR THE LEFT VENTRICLE AND AORTA?

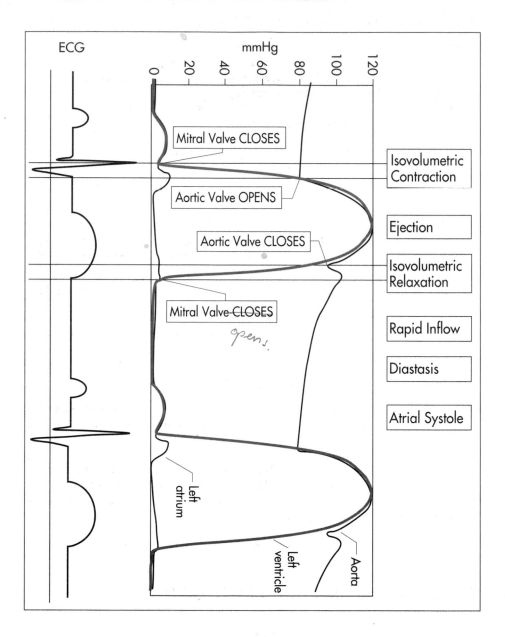

20. WHAT ARE THE CARDIOVASCULAR EFFECTS OF TILTING?

➡ **This tilting could be head up or head down.**

Head up tilt:
- There will be decreased cardiac return because of venous pooling.
- The muscle pump in the legs increases venous return, in the awake patient.
- Carotid sinus firing is reduced and this causes:
  - ➤ Compensatory tachycardia.
  - ➤ Increased sympathetic tone and vasoconstriction.

The result is increased heart rate and elevated blood pressure.
This response is reduced or abolished in:
  1. Autonomic neuropathy.
  2. Anaesthesia.

Head down tilt:
- There is increased venous return; some call this "autotransfusion".
- This increased preload causes increased cardiac output, by Starling's law of the heart.

But cardiac failure may occur in head-down tilting in fixed output states and fluid overload.

....

21. WHAT IS AUTOREGULATION OF BLOOD FLOW?

➡ **Autoregulation is the ability of an organ to control its blood supply independently of neural and hormonal influence. There are two mechanisms whereby it is mediated.**

  1. A fall in arterial pressure results in a reduction in blood flow, and accumulation of metabolites; these cause local terminal arteriolar dilation which increases flow.
  2. Myogenic response: This involves local neural reflexes in response to stretch, at the level of the 1st order arteriole.

....

22. WHAT IS THE EJECTION FRACTION OF LEFT VENTRICLE?

$$\text{Ejection fraction} = \frac{\text{Stroke Volume}}{\text{Left Ventricular End Diastolic Volume}}$$

- Measure by Doppler at echocardiography
- Normal >0.6. or 60%

....

23. WHAT IS STARLING'S LAW OF THE HEART?

➡ **Starling's law of the heart states that stroke volume is proportional to left ventricular end diastolic volume, to pressure, and to the length of the myofibril, therefore:**

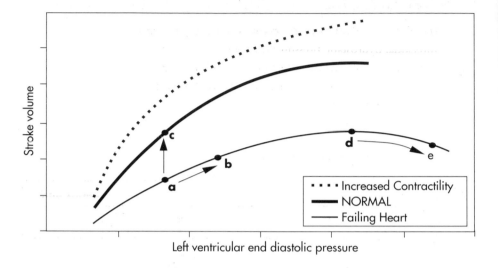

Left ventricular end diastolic pressure

This change of output due to change in fibre length is also known as heterometric regulation, as opposed to homometric regulation which is change in output due to altered contractility. The implication of the shape of the curves is that the failing heart will generate less stroke volume for the same end–diastolic volume.

Starling originally stated that **"the energy of contraction [of a myofibril] is proportional to the initial length of the cardiac muscle fiber"** *(sic)*.

This has been extrapolated to imply that the stroke volume is proportional to the end diastolic volume. If the compliance of the heart is assumed to be constant then the stroke volume is proportional to the end diastolic pressure. If the mitral valve is functioning normally then the end diastolic pressure is the same as the left atrial pressure. The object of a pulmonary capillary wedge pressure reading is to record the pressure in the pulmonary venous system and therefore in the left atrium by using a static column of blood to transmit the pressure to the transducer. Therefore the stroke volume may be proportional to the pulmonary capillary wedge pressure. However it can be seen that what is an excellent theory in the laboratory requires considerable faith in its application to the patient. It is also a mistake to assume that the CVP is consistently related to the stroke volume or to blood pressure.

Changes in the left ventricular end diastolic pressure ("preload") e.g. by altering the circulating volume, lead to shifts along one particular line (**a** to **b**), whereas changes in the contractility of the heart (e.g. by use of inotropic drugs) lead to a change of line (**a** to **c**). Therefore it can be seen that in the impaired myocardium a change in preload has a smaller effect than in the normal heart and can rapidly lead to the point where an increase in preload leads to a decrease in contractility (**d** to **e**).

••••••••••••••••••••••••••••••••

24. WHAT ARE THE STARLING FORCES IN CAPILLARIES, AND WHAT HAPPENS TO THEM IF 500ml BLOOD IS LOST?

➡️ **The forces are both hydrostatic and osmotic. You must be able to describe this diagram.**

P_c Capillary hydrostatic pressure (varies from artery to vein)

P_{if} Interstitial hydrostatic pressure (usually 0)

π_p Oncotic pressure due to plasma proteins (28 mmHg)

π_{if} Oncotic pressure due to interstitial proteins (3 mmHg)

(Osmotic = hydrostatic and oncotic)

$$\text{Net filtration} = (P_c - P_{if}) - (\pi_p - \pi_{if})$$

       ↑   ↑   ↑   ↑

     varies   constant   constant   constant

Arterial end   **Venous end**

$\pi_p = 28$ $\pi_p = 28$

$\pi_{if} = 3$ $P_c = 15$ mmHg $\pi_{if} = 3$

$P_c = 35$ mmHg

PRESSURE = (35-0) - (28-3)
= 35-25
= 10 mm Hg **OUT** of capillary

PRESSURE = (15-0) - (28-3)
= 15-25
= 10 mm Hg **INTO** capillary

If the patient loses 500ml of blood acutely, then the capillary hydrostatic pressure (P_c) falls especially at the venous end. The net pressure into the capillary increases and the balance is no longer maintained so fluid is retrieved into the circulation from the interstitium until P_c is restored. Note that this will also lead to small changes in π_p and π_{if}.

· ·

25. WHAT KEEPS ALVEOLI DRY?

➡️ **The fact that the capillary hydrostatic pressure is much lower on the right side of the circulation than on the left.**

Oedema will develop when:

1. P_c increases (this is a consequence of left ventricular failure).
2. π_p falls (in hypoalbuminaemia and fluid crystalloid overload).
3. Permeability increases (in acute lung injury and anaphylaxis).

· ·

26. WHAT CARDIORESPIRATORY CHANGES OCCUR IN PREGNANCY?

➡️ **There are changes in the circulatory volume, the cardiac output, and the pattern and depth of respiration.**

1. Increased circulatory volume:
   - Increased red cell mass by 20% (an action of erythropoeitin).
   - Increased plasma volume by 50% (due to NaCl and water retention).

2. Increased cardiac output: by 60% at 28 weeks
   - Increase in heart rate by 15%.
   - Increase in stroke volume by 30%.
   - Reduced systemic vascular resistance, so creating a tendency to vascular engorgement.
   - Mean arterial pressure stays constant.
   - Increase in glomerular filtration rate by 50%.

3. Increased ventilation: Alveolar ventilation increases by 70% at term.
   - Reduced $PaCO_2$.
   - Increased tidal volume.
   - Reduction in FRC by 20%.
   - Increased A-a DO_2, thus more rapid development of acidosis and hypoxia.

••••••••••••••••••••••••••••••

27. WHAT ARE THE CHANGES IN THE FOETAL CIRCULATION AT BIRTH?

➡️ **The key is the change in pressures induced by the sudden change in pulmonary vascular resistance**

Prior to birth:

Pulmonary vascular resistance is high because the lungs are not inflated. Blood from the right side of the heart, rather than go into the pulmonary arteries, goes into the ductus arteriosus and into the aorta, or through the foramen ovale and into the left atrium - because the **pressure on the right side exceeds the pressure on the left.**

At first gasp:

The lungs inflate and the pulmonary vascular resistance falls. There is suddenly a reduction in right-sided pressure and **so the pressure on the left side now exceeds the pressure on the right.**

As a result in the pressure change:
   - The foramen ovale closes.
   - Oxygenated blood flows retrograde in the ductus arteriosus.

As a result of this change:
   - The ductus arteriosus closes (but if cyanosed this fails to happen).

••••••••••••••••••••••••••••••

28. HOW DOES CORONARY BLOOD FLOW ALTER DURING THE CARDIAC CYCLE?

➡ **Coronary flow occurs in diastole (because intramyocardial vessels are compressed in systole) and is proportional to metabolic activity; in this way the system autoregulates.**

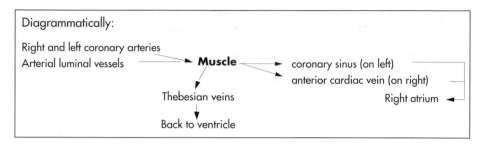

Flow at rest is 250 ml/min.

Myocardial O_2 consumption is 11 ml/100g tissue/min (for skeletal muscle it is 8 ml/100g tissue/min)

Coronary venous pO_2 is very low, so increased demand cannot be met by increased extraction – increased flow is required.

So: Increased heart rate ➡ decreased diastolic time ➡ decreased supply.

Increased intraventricular pressure ➡ decreased supply.

The pressure compresses vessels, decreasing supply, which happens in hypertensives and is one reason why they are susceptible to myocardial ischaemia.

●●●●●●●●●●●●●●●●●●●●●●●●●●●●●●●

29. WHAT ARE PORTAL CIRCULATIONS?

➡ **A portal circulation is one which connects two capillary beds but does not receive a direct arterial supply nor drain into a venous system.**

There are two of significance:

• The hepatic portal vein, connecting the alimentary tract and the liver. It conveys blood containing nutrients as well as toxins, and the liver converts the nutrients for storage or usage and metabolises the toxins. The hepatic portal circulation is vulnerable to a number of pathological processes, but if portal blood enters the systemic circulation, confusion, delirium or hepatic coma may ensue as toxins reach the central nervous system. In cirrhosis portal hypertension may result, with distension of veins which form part of the circulation. Those which lie in the lower part of the oesophagus are vulnerable to trauma and represent a common source of upper gastro-intestinal bleeding, which may be catastrophic in extreme cases.

• Hypothalamic - pituitary circulation. This conveys blood between the hypothalamus and the anterior pituitary. The arterial source is from the carotid arteries and the circle of Willis which form the primary plexus on the ventral surface of the hypothalamus. Capillaries drain into vessels which travel down the pituitary stalk and end in the pituitary capillaries. The hormones transiting this circulation are:

1. Thyrotropin releasing hormone (TRH)
2. Corticotropin releasing hormone (CRH)
3. Gonadotropin releasing hormone (GnRH)
4. Prolactin releasing hormone (PRH)
5. Prolactin inhibiting hormone (PIH)
6. Growth hormone releasing hormone (GRH)
7. Somatostatin

••••••••••••••••••••••••••••••••

30. WHAT IS THE DISTINCTION BETWEEN THE HAEMOGLOBIN AND THE MYOGLOBIN OXYGEN DISSOCIATION CURVES?

➡ **The myoglobin oxygen dissociation curve lies to the left of the haemoglobin dissociation curve which means that there is a tendency for haemoglobin to offload oxygen to myoglobin.**

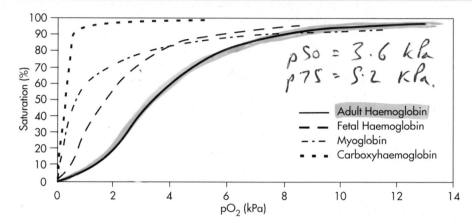

$p\,So = 3.6\ kPa$

$p\,7S = S.2\ kPa.$

—— Adult Haemoglobin
— — Fetal Haemoglobin
— · — Myoglobin
■ ■ ■ Carboxyhaemoglobin

1. Oxygen binding to haemoglobin is co-operative
2. O_2 - haemoglobin affinity is pH dependant whereas O_2 - myoglobin is not
3. O_2 - haemoglobin affinity is affected by 2,3 DPG.

The combined effect of the above mean that haemoglobin has a lower affinity for O_2 than has myoglobin.

Or, as a Hill plot:

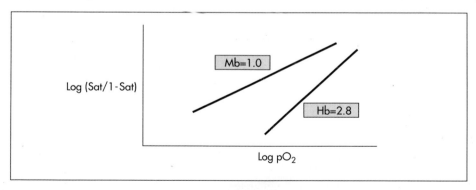

The fact that the Hill Coefficient for haemoglobin is greater than 1.0 means that the binding of O_2 to haemoglobin is co-operative.

So:

- Binding of O_2 at one tetramer facilitates binding at another.
- Unloading of O_2 at one tetramer facilitates unloading at another.

· ·

31. WHAT IS THE RESPONSE TO SUDDEN INCREASE IN ALTITUDE?

➡ **This is about decompression at altitude. If sudden, this will be observed:**

- Cold; temperature at 25,000 feet is usually -30°C. This is governed by the lapse rate, which is a drop in temperature of 1.98°C /1,000 feet.
- Misting. This is because of the dew point. There is an upper limit to the amount of water vapour air can hold at any temperature; when this maximum is reached the air is said to be saturated. Saturated air at high temperatures holds more water vapour than saturated air at low temperatures. The temperature at saturation is called the dew point. When decompression occurs, there is a sudden drop in temperature, but the same percentage of the air in the cabin is composed of water vapour, (even though the absolute quantity is reduced - but for the purposes of humidity it is percentages which matter) so the dew point is reached, and misting occurs.
- Hypoxia if above 8,000 feet. Alveolar air very rapidly equilibrates with the new ambient conditions. Pulmonary capillary blood will actually yield oxygen to the alveoli, in the opposite sense to normal, further accelerating the problem. This means that arterial oxygen tension falls very rapidly, depending on the severity of the decompression, with similarly rapid onset of symptoms of hypoxia.
- There will be expansion of closed cavities, because decreased pressure leads to increased volume.

The clinical observation is of a lowering in PaO_2, with a simultaneous lowering of $PaCO_2$; this latter effect is because there is a need to hyperventilate to reduce CO_2 to "make room" for O_2 because:

$$PaO_2 = PIO_2 - \frac{PACO_2}{R}$$

This contrasts with the effect of breathing a hypoxic gas mixture, which would be a question about the normal hypercapnia drive to ventilation and the fact that confusion, discoordination and ultimately unconsciousness occur before any profound dyspnoea is evident.

• •

32. WHAT COMPENSATION OCCURS IN CHRONIC ANAEMIA?

1. There is reduced blood viscosity, therefore there is increased cardiac output.
2. Increased 2, 3 DPG causes right-shifting of the oxyhaemoglobin dissociation curve, favouring offloading of O_2.
3. There is increased erythropoetin production.

• •

33. WHAT IS THE RESPONSE TO HAEMORRHAGE?

➡ Consider the four different interlinked systems: cardiovascular response, pituitary response, renin–aldosterone–angiotensin, and endocrine response from sympathetic nervous system.

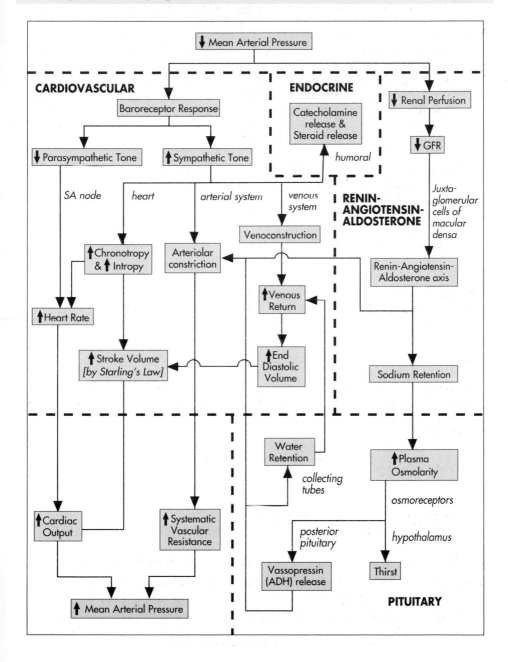

34. CAN YOU DESCRIBE THE VALSALVA MANOEUVRE?

➡ **The Valsalva manoeuvre is forced expiration against a closed glottis**

- There is an increase in intrathoracic pressure.
- There is therefore a drop in venous return.

The normal person maintains mean arterial pressure by:

- Increasing heart rate.
- Increasing systemic vascular resistance.
- And demonstrates, on release, transient hypertension and bradycardia.

There are four phases which can be drawn in a diagram:

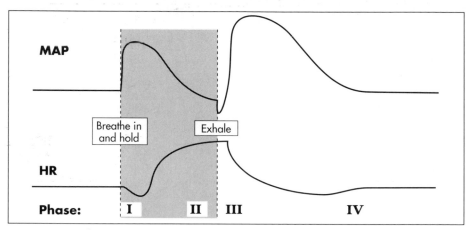

Phase I: The increase in intrathoracic pressure adds to arterial pressure producing a rise in mean arterial pressure.

Phase II: The mean arterial pressure then falls because of reduced venous return.

Phase III: On letting go, there is an overshoot as vasoconstriction and an increase in heart rate are still in operation.

Phase IV: Return to normal.

The Valsalva is absent or abnormal in autonomic dysfunction, in particular autonomic neuropathy (in diabetes mellitus, for example) and sympathectomy.

•••••••••••••••••••••••••••••••

35. CAN YOU DRAW THE CARDIAC ACTION POTENTIAL?

➡ **At rest, the membrane is more permeable to K⁺ than Na⁺ thus potential (Nernst equation) applies more to K⁺ (–90) than to Na⁺ (+60).**

➡ **It is the continuation of depolarisation which distinguishes cardiac action potential (AP) from skeletal AP. This is due to the action of slow Ca⁺⁺ channels, allowing Ca⁺⁺ entry into the cell, maintaining a balance against K⁺ outwards, so causing a prolonged depolarisation.**

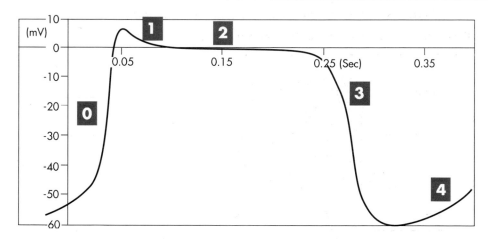

Phase:

    0 = Fast depolarisation, Na⁺ inwards.

    1 = Early incomplete repolarisation.

    2 = Plateau, slow Ca⁺⁺ inwards, prolonging AP.

    3 = Rapid repolarisation, K⁺ outwards.

    4 = Electrical diastole, refractory period.

Ca⁺⁺ is functionally related to β-receptors

K⁺ is functionally related to MII receptors and β-receptors

Changes in external K⁺ affect the resting potential level

Changes in internal Na⁺ affect the magnitude of the action potential

Effects on rate of firing:

Acetylcholine works at muscarinic (MII) receptors, causing increased K⁺ permeability (at special K⁺ channels), which in turn causes hyperpolarisation and decreased rate of firing.

Noradrenaline acts at β receptors to cause decreased K⁺ permeability and increased rate of firing. It also acts at β receptors causing increased Ca⁺⁺ permeability and increased strength of contraction.

•••••••••••••••••••••••••••••••

36. SO HOW DO ANTIARRHYTHMICS WORK?

VAUGHAN-WILLIAMS CLASSIFICATION

I a: Decreased Na^+ flux in phase 0; increased repolarisation; disopyramide
    b: Decreased Na^+ flux in phase 0; decreased repolarisation; lignocaine, mexilitine
    c: Decreased Na^+ flux in phase 0; flecainide

II: β-blockade; propranolol, metoprolol.

III: Enhanced repolarisation; bretylium, amiodarone

IV: Ca^{++} entry blockade; verapamil, nifedipine.

Recommendations for specific situations in adults:

- **VENTRICULAR ARRHYTHMIAS:**
  Lignocaine 100 mg then 2-4 mg/min, or mexilitine.

- **ATRIAL FIBRILLATION WITHOUT COMPROMISE:**
  Digoxin 1 mg divided in 24h, then 125-150 mcg/day; or DC SHOCK (start at 50J) after anticoagulation and stopping digoxin.

- **ATRIAL FIBRILLATION WITH COMPROMISE:**
  DC Shock.

- **FAST ATRIAL FIBRILLATION OF RECENT ONSET:**
  Flecainide 2 mg/kg then 1.5 mg/kg in one hour then 100-250 mcg/kg/hr.

- **WOOLF-PARKINSON-WHITE SYNDROME:**
  Amiodarone 5 mg/kg slow bolus then 200 mg/day.

- **LOCAL ANAESTHETIC TOXICITY:**
  Bretylium 7 mg/kg then 2 mg/min infusion.

- **OF RECENT ONSET:**
  Adenosine 3 mg, doubling until effect seen.

- **OTHER SUPRAVENTRICULAR TACHYCARDIA:**
  Verapamil 5 - 10 mg slow bolus.

- **TORSADES DES POINTES:**
  Magnesium 4 g bolus then infusion 1 g/hr, aim for 2 - 3.5 mmol/l.

·····························

37. WHAT ARE THE CAROTID BODIES AND SINUSES AND THEIR DIFFERENCES?

➡ **The carotid bodies are about oxygen; the carotid sinus is about pressure.**

Carotid (and aortic) bodies:

Contain two types of cell which are sensitive to **OXYGEN**

- Type I (Glomus) cells – adjacent to unmyelinated nerve endings from Glossopharyngeal nerve (IX). Dopamine exerts an inhibitory effect.
- Type II – sustentacular cells.

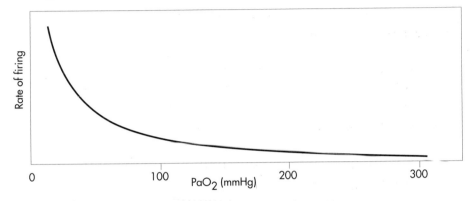

They receive a **colossal** arterial blood supply: 2 **litres**/100g tissue/minute. This means the glomus cells can function on supply from dissolved oxygen alone, and are unaffected by anaemia or CO poisoning.

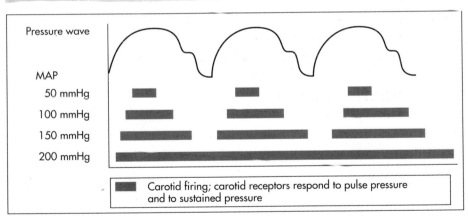

Carotid firing; carotid receptors respond to pulse pressure and to sustained pressure

Carotid Sinus:

This is situated at a dilatation of the internal carotid at its bifurcation, and is all about **PRESSURE**. Baroreceptors in dilatation resemble golgi tendon organs. The carotid sinus nerve is a branch of the glossopharyngeal (IX).

•••••••••••••••••••••••••••••••

38. WHY IS IT DESIRABLE FOR A PATIENT'S HAEMOGLOBIN TO EXCEED 10G/DL FOR ANAESTHESIA?

➡ **It has been traditional for patients to have a haemoglobin >10 g/dl for elective surgery.**

This is due to concerns for myocardial supply. The myocardium extracts 12 ml/dl of oxygen from every 100 ml of blood delivered to the coronary circulation. The CaO_2 of blood with a Hb of 10 g/dl is:

$(1.31 \times Hb \times Saturation/100) + 0.02\ pO_2$; assume blood to be 100% saturated and the FiO_2 to be 0.3, i.e. a safe anaesthetic;

$CaO_2 = (1.31 \times 10) + 0.02 \times \text{15}\ \ \text{30}$

$CaO_2 = 13.1 + 0.3$ $0.02\ kO_2$ ml/dl per kPa

$CaO_2 = 13.4$ ml/dl.

This comfortably exceeds the maximum extraction from the myocardial supply, and this is the reason why the rule applies.

....

39. WHAT IS ARTERIO-VENOUS O_2 DIFFERENCE?

➡ **This is the difference in <u>oxygen tension</u> between the arterial and venous circulations, reflecting the oxygen consumption of an organ or of the whole body.**

- O_2 content $= 1.31 \times (Hb \times Sat/100) + 0.02\ PaO_2$.
- $S\bar{v}O_2$ may be measured by a photometric cell at the pulmonary artery catheter tip (and thus $C\bar{v}O_2$ may be calculated from the above).
- PaO_2 can be measured directly from an arterial sample, and arterial O_2 calculated as above.
- Q, cardiac output, may be obtained from calorimetric measurement.

This allows calculation of $\dot{V}O_2$, oxygen consumption, from

Fick $\dot{Q} = \dfrac{\dot{V}O_2}{CaO_2 - C\bar{v}O_2}$

Diminished $\dot{V}O_2$ is the earliest pathophysiological event in shock, and usually precedes the hypotension that characterises it.

....

40. CAN YOU DRAW THE PRESSURES SEEN WHEN A PULMONARY ARTERY FLOTATION CATHETER (PAFC) IS INSERTED?

➡ Remember not to refer to a 'Swan–Ganz' catheter or to the placement of a PAFC as 'Swanning' or 'Ganzing'.

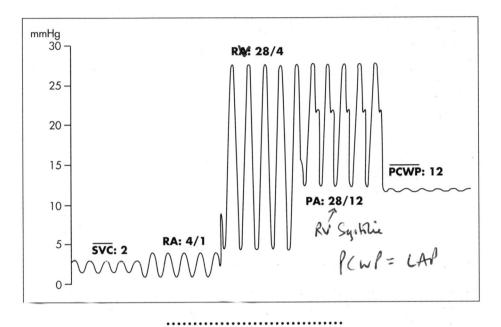

RV: 28/4

PCWP: 12

PA: 28/12

RV Systolic

PCWP = LAP

RA: 4/1

SVC: 2

· ·

41. WHAT ARE THE ACUTE CARDIOVASCULAR EFFECTS OF INTERMITTENT POSITIVE PRESSURE VENTILATION (IPPV)?

➡ Normal intrathoracic pressure is negative; this is reversed during IPPV, rather like a series of Valsalva manoeuvres which summate.

1. Venous return is impeded by the positive phase of IPPV.

2. There is a degree of cardiac tamponnade due to the inflation of the lungs.

3. There is increased pulmonary vascular resistance due to compression of the pulmonary capillaries.

4. Autonomic reflexes increase venous and arterial tone to compensate; however this may be ineffective in the compromised patient if there is deep anaesthesia, hypovolaemia, sympathetic blockade or ischaemic heart disease.

↑ ADH Secretion ·

3 QUESTIONS IN RESPIRATORY PHYSIOLOGY

1. CAN YOU DRAW THE OXYHAEMOGLOBIN DISSOCIATION CURVE?

➡ **If you cannot, you will fail.**

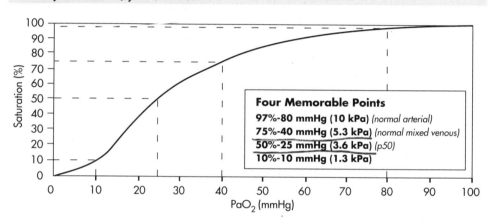

Four Memorable Points

97%-80 mmHg (10 kPa) *(normal arterial)*
75%-40 mmHg (5.3 kPa) *(normal mixed venous)*
50%-25 mmHg (3.6 kPa) *(p50)*
10%-10 mmHg (1.3 kPa)

By using the outdated mmHg there are four easily memorable points that help draw the curve. At the very least the three physiologically crucial points must be known:

Arterial	100% Saturated	PO$_2$ <12kPa
Mixed venous	75% saturated	PO$_2$ 5.3kPa
P50	50% saturated	PO$_2$ 3.6kPa

· ·

2. CAN YOU DERIVE THE BOHR EQUATION?

➡ **The Bohr equation allows derivation of total (physiological) dead space.**

1. $V_{D,Phys} = V_{D,Anat} + V_{D,Alv}$

2. V_A = volume of alveoli. F_{ACO_2} = Fraction of alveolar gas that is CO_2
   V_D = volume of dead space. F_{ECO_2} = Fraction of expired gas that is CO_2
   Tidal Volume, $V_T = V_D + V_A$

3. All CO_2 comes from alveoli (V_A) and none from dead space (V_D).

(Like the shunt equation, use total gas expired).

$$V_T \times F_{ECO_2} = \text{total } CO_2 \text{ "Flux" by analogy; collect in bag and measure}$$

Which all comes from

$$= V_A \times F_{ACO2}$$

4. $\qquad V_T \quad = V_A + V_D.$

Therefore $V_A \quad = V_T - V_D.$

5. Substitute 3 into 4.

$$V_T \times F_{ECO2} = (V_T - V_D) \times F_{ACO2}$$

6. Expand

$$V_T \times F_{ECO2} = (V_T \times F_{ACO2}) - (V_D \times F_{ACO2})$$

7. Add, so as to get V_T on one side

$$V_D \times F_{ACO2} = (V_T \times F_{ACO2}) - (V_T - F_{ECO2})$$

8. Simplify right side

$$V_D \times F_{ACO2} = V_T \times (F_{ACO2} - F_{ECO2})$$

9. Rearrange

$$V_D/V_T = \frac{F_A CO_2 - F_E CO_2}{F_A CO_2}$$

10. Bohr $\quad \dfrac{V_D}{V_T} \quad = \dfrac{P_A CO_2 - P_E CO_2}{P_A CO_2}$

. . . .

3. HOW DO YOU MEASURE RESPIRATORY DEAD SPACE?

➡ **Dead space is that part of inspired gas which does not take part in gas exchange. It is divided into alveolar dead space, $V_{D,alv}$, which consists of unperfused alveoli, and anatomical dead space, $V_{D,anat}$, which consists of the conducting airways.**

Helium dilution allows measurement of TOTAL LUNG CAPACITY, from which you can derive residual volume and FRC, by using spirometry and arithmetic. However it cannot measure that volume which is behind closed airways, because the Helium cannot get there; so,

In order to measure FRC in, for example, a patient with emphysema and airway closure, the body plethysmograph must be used. This uses Boyle's law, P1 x V1 = P2 x V2.

Anatomical dead space can be measured by Fowler's method, slow exhalation after single breath of 100% O_2, monitoring Nitrogen concentration. Perpendicular through phase II locates $V_{D, anat}$

$$V_{D, phys} = V_{D,alv} + V_{D,anat}$$

For $V_{D, phys}$, the Bohr equation: $$\frac{V_D}{V_T} = \frac{P_ACO_2 - P_ECO_2}{P_ACO_2}$$

For $V_{D,anat}$, Single breath O_2

The dead space is the volume up to the vertical line, placed so that the areas X and Y are equal.

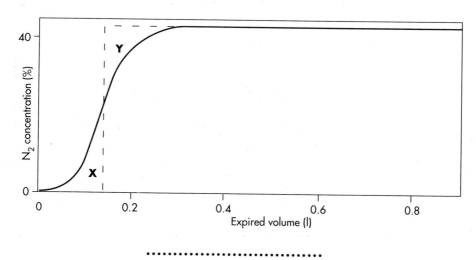

....

Helium dilution
Before equilibration

$$C_1 \times V_1 = C_2 \times (V_1 + V_2)$$

4. WHAT ARE THE FUNCTIONS OF THE NOSE?

➡ **This has been asked in the exam as a prelude to discussing humidification.**

1. Warming of inspired gases to within 3°C of body temperature.
2. Humidification of inspired gases to within 2% of saturated vapour pressure.
3. Filtration of particles from inspired gases.
4. Olfaction by first cranial nerve via cribriform plate.
5. Vocalisation by resonance of nasal sinuses.
6. Provision of dead space.

....

5. WHAT ARE THE EFFECTS OF HYPERCARBIA?

➡ **Hypercarbia is defined as a $PaCO_2$ greater than 45 mmHg (6.0 kPa). You should divide your answer into discussion of effects on each system in turn.**

• Effects on the central nervous system: Elevated CO_2 raises cerebral blood flow due to increased $[H^+]$. This effect only lasts until bicarbonate buffering becomes effective, at about 24 – 48 hours. Hypercarbia stimulates the sympathetic nervous system.
• Effects on the respiratory system: Elevation of CO_2 up to 100 mmHg (13.0 kPa) stimulates respiration, beyond that point it is a respiratory depressant. It also increases pulmonary vascular resistance.

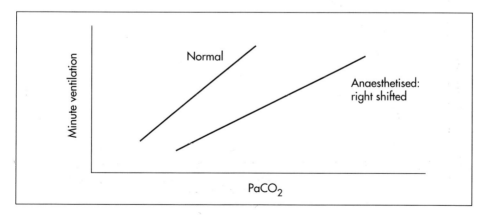

• Effects on the cardiovascular system: CO_2 is a direct myocardial depressant and a potent vasodilator. This effect is blunted at modest levels of hypercarbia because of the consequent sympathetic stimulation; more severe rises result in a fall in cardiac output and BP.

....

6. WHAT FACTORS AFFECT PULMONARY VASCULAR RESISTANCE?

➡ **Consider factors which increase pulmonary vascular resistance (PVR) and those which reduce it.**

Factors increasing pulmonary vascular resistance:

- A reduction in alveolar PO_2, which is known as hypoxic pulmonary vasoconstriction. This is a protective mechanism, which should divert blood away from locally under-ventilated areas. The effect is probably mediated by a fall in nitric oxide (NO).
- A rise in CO_2 and acidosis.
- Adrenaline, dopamine, histamine, serotonin.
- Lung collapse.

Factors reducing pulmonary vascular resistance:

- Increased cardiac output by recruitment of capillaries.
- Acetylcholine and cholinergics, possibly also an NO effect.
- Isoprenaline.
- Prostacyclin.

• •

7. HERE IS AN ARTERIAL BLOOD GAS SAMPLE, SHOWING ELEVATED CO_2 WITH LOW O_2. CAN YOU INTERPRET IT?

➡ **You may be given a blood gas result to comment on.**

High CO_2 with low O_2 implies type II respiratory failure: an exhausted asthmatic, for example.

- PCO_2 is related to ventilatory function and minute ventilation.
- PO_2 is related to gas exchange and inspired oxygen fraction.

Low pH and low PO_2 implies tissue acidosis. It is possible to differentiate acute from chronic hypoventilation by pH;

- Acute = acidotic, **NORMAL** bicarbonate.
- Compensated = normal pH, **HIGH** bicarbonate

• •

8. WHAT IS THE ALVEOLAR - ARTERIAL O_2 GRA

➡ **This is the difference between the observed arterial O_2 co**
calculated ideal alveolar O_2 content.

It may be calculated by subtracting the arterial PO_2 (measured) from the ideal alveolar PO_2, which may be calculated from:

$$P_AO_2 = P_IO_2 - \frac{P_ACO_2}{R}$$

The gradient is normally less than 2 kPa and is increased in disease states:
1. Left-to-right vascular shunt.
2. Ventilation/perfusion defects.
3. Diffusion impairment: extravascular lung water, pulmonary fibrosis, etc.
4. Adult respiratory distress syndrome.
5. Neonatal respiratory distress syndrome.

....

9. WHAT IS THE OXYGEN CASCADE?

➡ **The oxygen cascade describes the drop in oxygen tension between**
atmospheric air and the surface of the mitochondrion.

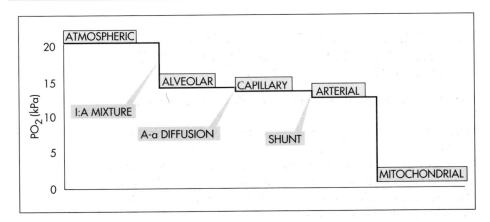

....

43

J. WHAT IS PULMONARY VENOUS ADMIXTURE?

➡ **Venous admixture equals true shunt plus $\dot{V}/\dot{Q}$ mismatch.**

From the 'shunt' equation $\quad \dfrac{\dot{Q}s}{\dot{Q}_T} = \dfrac{CiO_2 - CaO_2}{CiO_2 - C\bar{v}O_2}$

$\dot{Q}s/\dot{Q}_T$ is the ratio of 'shunt' to total cardiac output

- CaO_2
- $C\bar{v}O_2$

require arterial and mixed venous samples (from a pulmonary artery catheter) and this calculation:

O_2 content = (1.31 x Hb x Saturation/100) + 0.02 PO_2

True shunt:

- This is due to bronchial blood flow emerging from the bronchial veins; it represents 5% of cardiac output in normal states.

$\dot{V}/\dot{Q}$ mismatch: this is about the West zones.

- Apices are ventilated better than perfused;
- Midzones "normal", i.e. $P_a > P_A > P_v$
- Bases perfused better than ventilated.
- When $P_A > P_a > P_v$ (apices) there is no perfusion.

Ratio of V:Q totals at 1.0 : 0.8

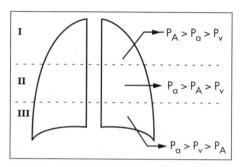

$$P_A > P_a > P_v$$
$$P_a > P_A > P_v$$
$$P_a > P_v > P_A$$

· ·

11. WHAT NON-RESPIRATORY FUNCTIONS OF THE LUNGS DO YOU KNOW?

1. Removal of vasoactive amines and neurotransmitters, which is a function of pulmonary endothelial cells.
2. Metabolism of Angiotensin I to Angiotensin II, which is a vasopressor and a part of the stress response.
3. Filtration of peripheral venous blood of clots, etc.
4. Phospholipid synthesis, e.g. dipalmitoyl phosphatidyl choline which is a component of surfactant.
5. Prostaglandin inactivation.
6. Leukotriene synthesis (from arachidonic acid, which is lipoxygenase mediated).
7. Immunoglobulin synthesis; IgA.

· ·

12. WHAT IS WHOLE BODY O_2 CONSUMPTION?

➡ $\dot{V}O_2 = C(a-\bar{v})\ O_2$ x cardiac index x 10.

Normal $= 100 - 180$ ml/min/m^2

••••••••••••••••••••••••••••••

13. CAN YOU DRAW THE VOLUMES AND CAPACITIES OF THE LUNG?

➡ **A capacity consists of TWO or more volumes.**

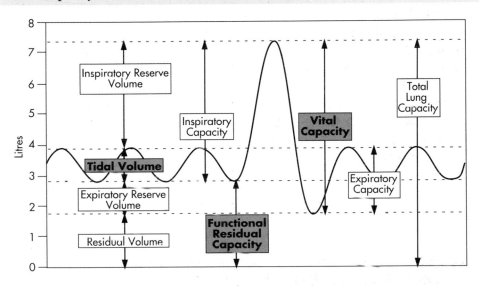

All figures refer to the adult.

Tidal volume: The volume of gas in a normal resting respiration. (500ml or 7ml/kg).

Vital capacity: The maximum amount of gas which can be used in one breath, made up of IRV and ERV in addition to TV.(4.5 l).

Total lung capacity: 7.5 l.

Functional residual capacity: An area of respiratory physiology of supreme interest to anaesthetists. This is the amount of gas in the lungs after a normal tidal breath. It is where the gas is exchanged, and is reduced by anaesthesia. The significance of this is in the following:

Closing Capacity = Closing Volume + Residual Volume: Closing Capacity is the volume of the lungs at which small airways start to close and rises with age. FRC is reduced by 20% in anaesthesia due to diaphragmatic shift, decreased ribcage dimensions and IPPV. If FRC falls below Closing Capacity, areas will be perfused but not ventilated.

••••••••••••••••••••••••••••••

14. HOW ARE THE ALVEOLAR PARTIAL PRESSURES OF CO$_2$ AND O$_2$ RELATED?

➡️ **The O$_2$ - CO$_2$ diagram shows the ventilation-perfusion ratio line.**

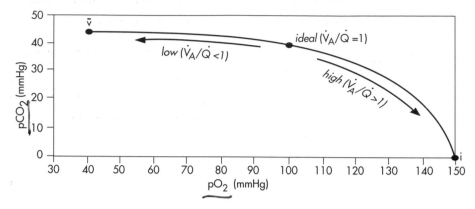

The oxygen and CO$_2$ composition of the blood are not independent, but related by means of this line. This shows all possible alveolar gas compositions for a lung with inspired fraction of I, in this case 20 kPa, and the effects of increased and decreased $\dot{V}/\dot{Q}$ ratios.

....

15. WHY IS IT USUAL TO USE 30% O$_2$ DURING ANAESTHESIA?

➡️ **This is a popular question which has a simple answer, but which then provides the opportunity to explore one of the three main causes of hypoxia under anaesthesia.**

➡️ **To compensate for the relative hypoxia which would otherwise occur under general anaesthesia, due to:**

1. Ventilation-perfusion mismatch, which occurs under anaesthesia because of closing capacity encroaching on FRC.
2. Hypoventilation, with reduced respiratory rate and reduced tidal volume.
3. Abolition of hypoxic pulmonary vasoconstriction (HPV) by volatile anaesthetic agents. HPV normally confers a protective influence by reducing perfusion of poorly-oxygenated areas of the lungs; this is lost under anaesthesia.

....

16. CAN YOU DESCRIBE THE RISE IN P_AO_2 WHEN BREATHING 100% O_2?

➡ **This is about preoxygenation (denitrogenation), and the fact that the SVP of water vapour is 47 mmHg, applies to alveolar gas, and is independent of atmospheric pressure but does depend on temperature.**

It is NOT the same as the time taken for the SpO_2 to reach 100%.

For the whole body to be denitrogenated, the process proceeds at an exponential rate and takes several hours.

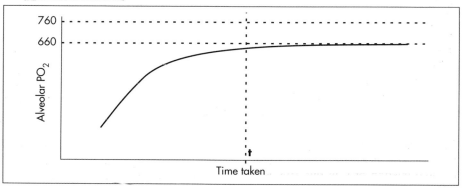

t, the time taken to equilibrium, is normally 10 minutes, but is affected by:

1. Health.
2. Chronic airways disease, which increases t.
3. Cardiac output, where a low output increases t.

Most would advocate preoxygenation for 3-5 minutes, or for three vital capacity breaths. Water vapour occupies 47 mmHg and CO_2 40 mmHg, hence optimal alveolar O_2 at normal ventilation breathing 100% O_2 is around 660 mmHg.

•••••••••••••••••••••••••••••••

17. WHAT IS CHEST COMPLIANCE?

➡ **Compliance is the change in volume per unit change in pressure.**

$$1/c_{TOTAL} = 1/c_{LUNG} + 1/c_{CHEST\ WALL}$$

Why reciprocals? Because pressure at a given volume is inversely proportional to compliance.

Compliance decreases with

- Venous congestion
- Oedema
- Intermittent positive pressure ventilation
- Fibrosis, emphysema
- Age

•••••••••••••••••••••••••••••••

18. CAN YOU DESCRIBE RESPIRATION IN THE NEONATE?

➡ **This can be divided into anatomical and physiological considerations.**

Anatomical:
- Neonates have a large head, a short neck, and a proportionally large tongue.
- They have narrow passages.
- They are nasal breathers; the epiglottis touches the soft palate.
- Their larynx is high, and narrowest at the cricoid, which is at the level of C3-4.
- The epiglottis is bigger in proportion, and it is U-shaped.
- There is a wider carina than in older children, and both main bronchi are at equal angles.
- There are 21 generations of airway.
- There are 10% of the number of adult alveoli.

Physiological:
- High compliance, small functional residual capacity (FRC).
- The closing volume added to the residual volume = closing capacity (CC); CC is greater than FRC until aged 5, which implies a tendency to airway closure and V/Q mismatch.
- Tidal volume is fixed because of:
    - Horizontal ribs.
    - Weak intercostal muscles.
    - Large abdomen.

So, in order to increase minute volume ($\dot{V}_E$), neonates need to increase respiratory rate (which is analogous to the situation with cardiac output in the neonate, where stroke volume is fixed, and rate dictates output).

- Respiratory rate is 32 breaths per minute in the neonate; to calculate aged 1-13, = (24-age/2) per minute
- Minute volume ~ 200 ml/Kg body weight ⎱ So for a 3kg neonate:
- Tidal volume ~ 8 ml/Kg body weight ⎰ $\dot{V}_E$ = 600 ml
    Tidal volume (V_T) = 20 ml
- A low PaO_2, and a low $PaCO_2$ are compatible with normality.
- There is no expiratory pause: The respiratory cycle is a sine wave.

....

19. HOW IS ALVEOLAR VENTILATION CONTROLLED?

➡ **Alveolar ventilation is proportional to rate of respiration and to depth of respiration.**

➡ **Discuss receptors, comparators, and effectors.**

Receptors: Those responding to CO_2 are the most significant in health.

1. Receptors for $PaCO_2$ are present in the ventrolateral medulla near the 9th and 10th cranial nerves. These receptors are surrounded by cerebrospinal fluid (CSF) and are responsive to $[H^+]$ ion concentration and therefore indirectly to the presence of CO_2 by means of the action of carbonic anhydrase. The CO_2 diffuses across the blood brain barrier, $[H^+]$ is generated and the receptors stimulated. CSF has fewer proteins than plasma, and hence less buffering ability - so pH changes are more pronounced.

2. The receptors for PaO_2 are the carotid and aortic bodies. The type I glomus cells demonstrate a linear response to $[H^+]$; they respond to $[O_2]$ in a non-linear fashion, firing only when the PaO_2 falls below 13 kPa. The carotid and aortic bodies receive an abundant blood supply, which allows for precise comparisons to be made as they have a very low arterio-venous O_2 difference despite having a high metabolic rate. They are relatively indifferent to $PaCO_2$.

3. Airway stretch receptors: These act to terminate respiration, by means of the Hering-Breuer reflex.

4. Epithelial receptors in the larynx: These respond to irritants and inhibit respiration.

5. J Receptors (meaning juxta-capillary) respond to capillary engorgement (as in pulmonary oedema) by inhibiting respiration. This may be an explanation for the dypnoea of pulmonary oedema.

Comparators: these are all under a degree of control by the cortex

1. The Nucleus Parabrachialis Medialis (NPBM) is located in the pons and is referred to as the pneumotactic centre. It fine-tunes respiration, influencing the other centres which are lower in the brainstem.

2. The inspiratory centre may be responsible for the intrinsic pattern of respiration.

3. The expiratory centre is only active during exercise, as it is only then that expiration becomes important; it is otherwise passive.

Effectors:

1. Diaphragm: Inspiratory function predominates, under phrenic innervation.

2. Intercostals: These are expiratory in function.

3. Accessory muscles: These are only used in extreme situations.

••••••••••••••••••••••••••••••••

20. HOW IS CO_2 TRANSPORTED IN THE BLOOD?

1. 60% as $HCO_3^- + H^+$ by means of carbonic anhydrase.
2. 30% as $HbCO_2$
3. 10% dissolved in plasma.

Resting production of CO_2 is 200 mls/minute.

$$\text{Respiratory quotient} \quad = \quad \frac{CO_2 \text{ produced}}{O_2 \text{ consumed}}$$

$$\text{usually} \quad = \quad 0.8$$

In Hb, combines with amino group

$$R\text{-}NH_2 \; + \; CO_2 \; \rightarrow \; R\text{-}\underset{\overset{|}{H}}{N}\text{-}COOH$$

Deoxyhaemoglobin has a higher affinity for both H^+ and CO_2 than does oxyhaemoglobin. This is the Haldane effect; thus O_2 deficient cells are better buffers than are oxygenated cells.

....

21. CAN YOU CLASSIFY HYPOXIA?

➡ **Hypoxia may be hypoxaemic, stagnant, cytotoxic or anaemic; after giving this definition, a discussion will follow on one of the four.**

1. **Hypoxaemic hypoxia;** where the PaO_2 is reduced, which may be due to:
   • Hypoventilation
   • Diffusion impairment
   • Shunt
   • $\dot{V}/\dot{Q}$ mismatch (N.B. not deadspace which is to do with CO_2)
2. **Stagnant hypoxia;** where the blood supply to an organ is inadequate, even though the PaO_2 and the Hb concentration may be normal.
3. **Cytotoxic hypoxia;** where the oxygen delivery is normal, but the cell is prevented from utilising it, for example, cytochrome poisoning.
4. **Anaemic hypoxia;** where the PaO_2 is normal but the Hb concentration, and therefore the amount of O_2 delivered, is deficient.

....

22. WHAT IS THE WORK OF BREATHING?

➡ This is the work required to move the lung and chest wall.

Work = pressure x volume. So, we need a pressure-volume curve to describe this phenomenon.

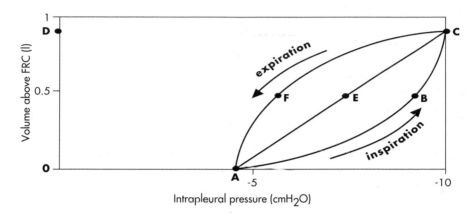

1. In inspiration the lung follows the line **ABC** and so the work done is described by the area **OABCDO** which is made up of:
   • **OAECDO** is the work required to overcome the elastic forces.
   • **ABCEA** is the work required to overcome the viscous (airway and tissue) resistance.

2. In expiration the area **AECFA** represents the work to overcome the airway (and tissue) resistance, and as this is within the area **OABCDO** it is accomplished by the stored energy within the elastic recoil that is released during passive expiration. The remaining part of the stored energy **OAFCDO**) is lost as heat.

In states of higher airway resistance or higher inspiratory flow rate **ABC** curves more to the right (that is there is a greater negative intrapleural pressure for a given volume) thus the viscous volume **ABCEA** is larger. Thus at higher ventilatory rates the viscous work of breathing is increased.

However with larger tidal volumes the elastic work area **OAECDO** is increased.

In patients with stiff lungs (thus reduced compliance) the elastic work is reduced by breathing with small tidal volumes at high respiratory rates (the so called 'pink puffer') , whereas in those patients with obstructive airway disease the viscous work is reduced by using a low respiratory rate, this the patients naturally find the respiratory pattern that ensures the lowest work of breathing.

$$\text{Efficiency} = \frac{\text{Useful work}}{\text{Energy expended}} \times 100$$

The efficiency of the work of breathing is usually about 5%; 5% is also the percentage of total O_2 consumption, at rest, used in the work of breathing.

• •

23. WHAT IS THE HENDERSON-HASSELBALCH EQUATION?

➡ **A buffer consists of weak acid with the conjugate base**

$$H^+ + A^- \underset{k_2}{\overset{k_1}{\rightleftharpoons}} HA \quad \text{at equilibrium, } k_1 = k_2$$

$$\frac{[H^+] \times [A^-]}{[HA]} = K \quad \text{by the law of mass action}$$

$$pH = pK + \log \frac{[HCO_3^-]}{0.2 \, PCO_2}$$ where 0.2 is the solubility coefficient of CO_2 in mmol/l/kPa.

It may usefully be simplified:

$$pH \, \alpha \, \frac{[HCO_3^-]}{[CO_2]}$$

Such that if the bicarbonate rises, or the CO_2 falls, then the pH will rise (an alkalosis will develop); by the same token, if the bicarbonate falls, or the CO_2 rises, the pH will fall; this is an acidosis.

• •

24. CAN YOU COMPARE THE DAVENPORT AND THE SIGGARD - ANDERSON DIAGRAMS?

➡ **Davenport plots plasma bicarbonate against pH, with PCO_2 lines on the graph allowing each defect, acidosis/alkalosis and respiratory/metabolic, to be shown as a vector. Siggard-Anderson plots log PCO_2 against pH, with a bicarbonate (buffer) curve on the graph. The lines are called "Isopleths".**

This is a simplification, but it is a reproducible version for the exam:

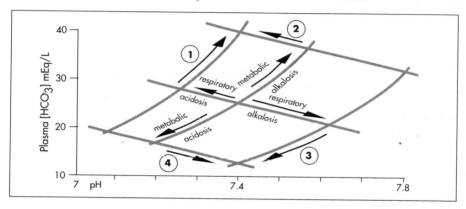

Compensation occurs towards the 7.4 line, i.e. renal H^+ excretion and HCO_3 retention as shown.

1 = Renal (metabolic) compensation for respiratory acidosis.
2 = Respiratory compensation for metabolic alkalosis.
3 = Renal (metabolic) compensation for respiratory alkalosis.
4 = Respiratory compensation for metabolic acidosis.

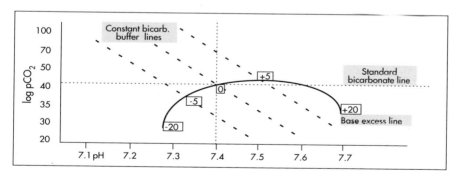

The standard bicarbonate line indicates the bicarbonate level for a $PaCO_2$ of 40 mmHg.

Siggard-Anderson was used before availability of the CO_2 electrode: A sample was equilibrated with known "low" gas and known "high" gas, a line was drawn and values read from the nomogram. The line is called the "buffer" line.

• •

25. CAN YOU DERIVE THE SHUNT EQUATION?

➡ **Need a diagram to do this.**

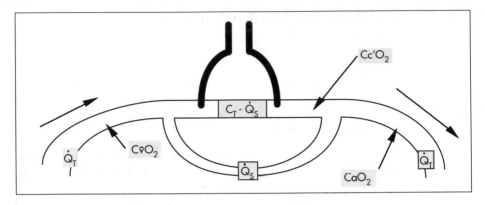

$\dot{Q}_T \times CaO_2$ = total oxygen flux from entire system

= that via shunt + that via alveolar capillary

= $\dot{Q}_S \times C\bar{v}O_2$ (that blood which doesn't get oxygenated at all)
$+ (\dot{Q}_T - \dot{Q}s) \times Cc'O_2$

Thus: $\dot{Q}_T \times CaO_2$ = $\dot{Q}_S \times C\bar{v}O_2$ + $(\dot{Q}_T - \dot{Q}_S) \times Cc'O_2$

Rearranging $\dfrac{\dot{Q}_S}{\dot{Q}_T}$ = $\dfrac{Cc'O_2 - CaO_2}{Cc'O_2 - C\bar{v}O_2}$

or $\dfrac{\dot{Q}_S}{\dot{Q}_T}$ = $\dfrac{C_iO_2 - CaO_2}{C_iO_2 - C\bar{v}O_2}$ (C_iO_2 is obtained from alveolar gas equation)

4 QUESTIONS IN ENDOCRINE PHYSIOLOGY

1. WHAT ARE THE FUNCTIONS OF THE POSTERIOR PITUITARY?

➡ **The posterior pituitary produces hormones which influence plasma osmolarity and circulating volume, milk ejection and uterine contraction.**

The posterior pituitary is the neurohypophysis. It is related to the hypothalamus via the hypothalamo–hypophyseal tract which lies within the hypophyseal stalk. It produces two peptide hormones, vasopressin (ADH, anti-diuretic hormone) and oxytocin, which are structually related.

Vasopressin:

```
        ┌──── S = S ────┐
Cys - Tyr - Phe - Gln - Asn - Cys - Pro - Arg - Gly - NH₂
```

Oxytocin:

```
        ┌──── S = S ────┐
Cys - Tyr - Ile - Gln - Asn - Cys - Pro - Leu - Gly - NH₂
```

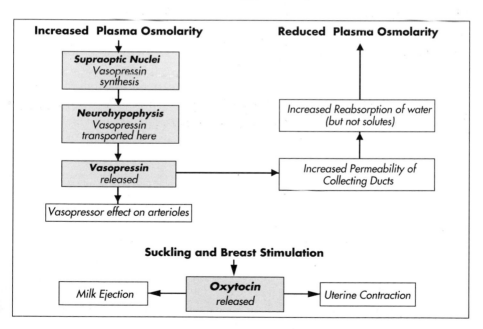

Increased Plasma Osmolarity

- **Supraoptic Nuclei** — Vasopressin synthesis
- **Neurohypophysis** — Vasopressin transported here
- **Vasopressin** released
- Vasopressor effect on arterioles

Reduced Plasma Osmolarity

- Increased Reabsorption of water (but not solutes)
- Increased Permeability of Collecting Ducts

Suckling and Breast Stimulation

- Milk Ejection ← **Oxytocin** released → Uterine Contraction

....

2. WHAT ARE THE FUNCTIONS OF ANTIDIURETIC HORMONE?

1. Antidiuretic hormone (ADH) causes increased distal nephron permeability to water. This results in greater retrieval of water from the distal nephron and less urine production.
2. Direct vasoconstriction.
   - Coronary
   - Splanchnic
   - Pulmonary
3. Smooth muscle contraction.
4. Stimulation of clotting factor production. This is an endothelial phenomenon.

....

3. HOW MAY HORMONAL SECRETION BE CONTROLLED?

1. By basal continuous secretion with negative feedback, e.g. thyroid hormones.
2. Secretion may be in response to:
   - Stress.
   - Blood parameters, e.g. insulin and glucagon, PTH and Calcium.
3. By time cycled rhythms:
   - Circadian rhythm, e.g. ACTH is highest in the morning.
   - Monthly rhythm, e.g. LH/FSH.

....

4. WHAT ARE THE FUNCTIONS OF THYROID HORMONE?

1. Sensitisation of myocardium to catecholamines; this is by β receptor synthesis.
2. Basal metabolic rate increase (possibly by Na/K-ATPase activity).
3. Reflexes and central nervous system (CNS) enhancement.
4. Growth Hormone facilitation.
5. CNS development.
6. Increased carbohydrate absorption (which increases plasma glucose after meals).
7. Lowering of plasma cholesterol.

Mechanism of action:

1. T_3 enters cells and binds nuclear receptors.
2. Hormone-receptor complex binds DNA, and increases expression of certain genes.
3. Messenger RNAs are formed; these are proteins which alter cellular function.

....

5. HOW IS THYROID HORMONE FORMED?

➡ **Thyroid hormone is formed in the thyroid gland from intestinally-absorbed iodine (in ionised form) and tyrosine, which is present as thyroglobulin.**

Tyrosine

$$HO-\bigcirc-CH_2-CH\begin{array}{c}NH_2\\|\\COOH\end{array}\quad\overset{+}{NH_2}$$

Oxidised iodine (I_3^- or I_0)
Iodinase

Monoiodotyrosine

Oxidised iodine (I_3^- or I_0)
Iodinase

Diiodotyrosine

condensation of two molecules
(under the influence of Thyroid Stimulation Hormone (TSH)

Thyroxine (T$_4$)

| If this Iodine is replaced by a Hydrogen atom then the molecule is **3,5',3' Tri-iodothyronine (T3)** *This is made by the reaction of diiodotyrosine and monoiodotyrosine* | If this Iodine is replaced by a Hydrogen atom then the molecule is **3,3',5' Tri-iodothyronine (rT3)** *This is probably inactive and may be produced in disease states to reduce energy consumption* |

TSH performs three functions:

1. It encourages the uptake of Iodine from the gut.
2. It converts diiodothyronine into thyroxine.
3. It causes the release of T_3 and T_4 into the blood.

. . . .

6. CAN YOU DISCUSS THE MAINTENANCE OF BODY TEMPERATURE?

➡ **Humans are homeotherms, with circadian rhythms. Temperature is highest during awake state and at ovulation. As before, we recommend that you discuss in the order of receptors–comparators–effectors.**

Receptors:

These are central and peripheral. The central receptors are the most important and actually regulate body temperature by influencing neural and hormonal changes. Peripheral receptors help by providing information on the how hot or cold the body part is, and so may influence behaviour.

- Central:
    Hypothalamus.
    Spinal cord.
    Abdominal viscera.
- Peripheral:
    Skin.
    Mucous membranes.

Comparator:

- Hypothalamus.

Effectors:

- Neuronal.
- Hormonal; T4, adrenaline.

Mechanisms increasing heat and causing heat preservation:

1. Vasoconstriction and piloerection.
2. Behavioural patterns: curl up, seek shelter, increase clothing.
3. Shivering, which generates heat but at considerable energy expense.
4. Increased activity.
5. Non-shivering thermogenesis; this takes place in brown fat, and is observed only in neonates.

Mechanisms decreasing heat and allowing for heat dissipation:

1. Vasodilatation.
2. Sweating; this is a cholinergic mediated function
3. Hyperventilation. Dogs hyperventilate dead space, eliminating heat, but not ventilating alveoli, which is why they don't pass out while panting.
4. Decreased activity.

....

7. HOW IS TEMPERATURE REGULATED IN A COLD ENVIRONMENT?

➡ **There are acute and chronic adjustments.**

Acclimatisation, after chronic exposure:
- Increase basal metabolic rate (BMR).
- Increase fat insulation.
- Reduce vasoconstrictor response to cold, which is a feature of Eskimo physiology.

Acute response:

1. Reduce heat loss: abolished by anaesthesia
   - Vasoconstriction.
   - Reduce surface area (curl up).
   - Behavioural: make shelter, dressing.

2. Increase heat production:
   - Increase muscle tone.
   - Shivering.
   - Non-shivering thermogenesis (brown fat).
   - Increased TSH, increased catecholamines.
   - Increased basal metabolic rate.
   - Increased appetite.

....

5 QUESTIONS IN GASTROINTESTINAL PHYSIOLOGY

1. CAN YOU DESCRIBE THE ACT OF SWALLOWING?

➡ **Up-back-shut-shut-swallow.**

Mastication puts a bolus on the dorsum of the tongue.

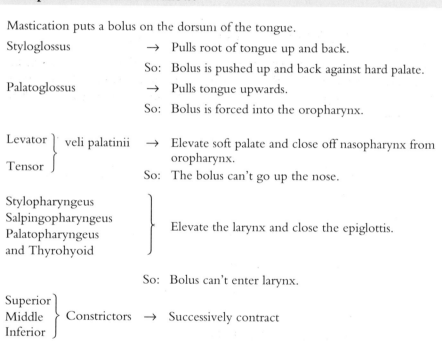

Styloglossus   →   Pulls root of tongue up and back.

     So: Bolus is pushed up and back against hard palate.

Palatoglossus   →   Pulls tongue upwards.

     So: Bolus is forced into the oropharynx.

Levator ⎫ veli palatinii   →   Elevate soft palate and close off nasopharynx from
Tensor ⎭   oropharynx.

     So: The bolus can't go up the nose.

Stylopharyngeus
Salpingopharyngeus   ⎫
Palatopharyngeus   ⎬   Elevate the larynx and close the epiglottis.
and Thyrohyoid   ⎭

     So: Bolus can't enter larynx.

Superior ⎫
Middle   ⎬ Constrictors   →   Successively contract
Inferior ⎭

     So: The bolus forced is into the oesophagus.

N.B. 1. Upper fibres of superior constrictor also help to occlude the nasopharynx.

      2. Lower fibres of inferior constrictor form the cricopharyngeus muscle.

•••••••••••••••••••••••••••••••

2. WHAT IS THE MECHANISM OF VOMITING?

➡ **Clear the route – squeeze – open – vomit.**

1. Deep breath.
2. Raise hyoid and larynx to pull cricoesophageal sphincter open;
3. Close glottis.
4. Elevation of soft palate to close off nasopharynx.
5. Contraction of diaphragm and abdominal muscles, raising intra–abdominal pressure.
6. Open gastro-oesophageal sphincter.

....

3. HOW IS LIVER BLOOD FLOW REGULATED?

➡ **The liver receives about 40% of cardiac output, 100 ml/100g tissue/min. It has a dual supply, 500 ml/min from the hepatic artery, which is 95% saturated, and 1000 ml/min from the hepatic portal vein, which is 70% saturated.**

Control is passive and active. Normal O_2 extraction is <50%, if demand increases extraction increases initially.

Active control is intrinsic or extrinsic; intrinsic depends on hepatic artery/hepatic portal vein reciprocity.

Extrinsic control:

- Sympathetics: These decrease liver blood flow and liver blood volume; this is a reservoir function;
- Drugs: Vasopressin: lowers portal pressure.

....

4. WHAT IS BARRIER PRESSURE?

➡ **Barrier pressure is lower oesophageal sphincter pressure (LOSP) minus intragastric pressure.**

If a pressure transducer were passed from oesophagus into stomach, a pattern would be observed. Initially, thoracic pressure is transmitted across the oesophageal wall, and varies with respiration. After the lower oesophageal sphincter, stomach pressure changes with gastric contractions and diaphragmatic movement.

The significance is that LOSP is reduced by pregnancy, drugs (atropine, suxamethonium) and that intragastric pressure is increased in the fed state. When one encroaches on the other, barrier pressure fails and reflux is possible.

....

5.   HOW IS FAT ABSORBED FROM THE GUT?

➡ **Fat is the same as triglyceride; the absorption is a two-stage process.**

➡ **Bile salts do two things.**

1. They cause emulsion of fat.
2. They act to form micelles in order to move the glyceride further down the gut.

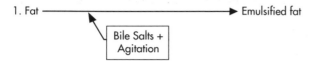

This is by reduction in surface tension of large globules, making small globules, then smaller globules, and finally an emulsion.

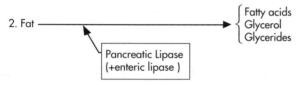

However the glycerides could re-combine with the fatty acids; but bile salts form the glycerides into micelles and move further down the lumen to be absorbed elsewhere, so that this does not happen.

· ·

6.   WHAT IS THE COMPOSITION AND FUNCTION OF BILE?

➡ **Bile is produced at 1-2 litres/day and has six main components:**

1. Bile salts
2. Cholesterol ⎫ these are synthesised in liver, and emulsify fat in the gut.
3. Lecithin

4. Bicarbonate ion; this neutralises gastric acid in the duodenum.

5. Bile pigments ⎫ these contribute to the elimination of metabolic products.
6. Trace metals

· ·

7. CAN YOU LIST THE FUNCTIONS OF THE LIVER?

1. Production of bile.
2. Excretion of bilirubin.
3. Storage of glucose as glycogen.
4. Formation of Acetoacetic acid from Acetyl CoA as end point of fatty acid metabolism.
5. Kupffer cells are part of the reticuloendothelial system, and cleanse portal venous blood.
6. Production of plasma proteins.
7. Production of clotting factors.
8. Formation of urea from ammonia.
9. Metabolism of drugs and toxins in two stages/phases.
   - Metabolism: oxidation/hydrolysis/sulphation.
   - Conjugation.
10. Blood reservoir.
11. Generation of heat.

There is a countercurrent mechanism at work. The hepatic sinusoid, which contains hepatic portal venous blood, flows in the opposite direction to the bile canaliculus.

••••••••••••••••••••••••••••••

8. WHAT ARE THE EFFECTS OF A TOTAL BILIARY FISTULA?

➡ **Gall bladder bile is ten times more concentrated than hepatic bile.**

1. Loss of fluid: 2 litres/day.
2. Acidosis: loss of bicarbonate.
3. Malabsorption of fats and fat soluble vitamins; A,D,E,K.
4. Steatorrhoea.

••••••••••••••••••••••••••••••

9. WHAT IS THE COMPOSITION OF GASTRIC JUICE, AND WHAT STIMULATES ITS PRODUCTION?

Composition:

Substance	Origin	Cellular source	Location
Acid : HCl : 2L/day	H+ATPase pump	Parietal cells	Body of Stomach
Pepsinogen: (→ Pepsin)	Protein synthesis	Chief cells	Body and Atrium
Mucus	Glycoprotein	Cells at top of gastric glands	Entirety of stomach

Production:

Phase	Mediating mechanisms	Result
Cephalic phase	Parasympathetics, gastrin	↑HCl
Gastric phase	Long and short neural reflexes, gastrin	↑HCl
Intestinal phase	Long and short neural reflexes, Secretin, Cholecystokinin	↓HCl

● ●

10. HOW IS GASTRIC EMPTYING MEASURED?

In order of how commonly the methods are employed:

1. By aspiration and direct measurement of residue by nasogastric or orogastric tube.
2. Solute absorption; commonly paracetamol uptake is measured, which only takes place after passage of the drug from the gastric lumen into the small intestine. This relies on the assumption that the difference in drug plasma concentration with time is due to difference in absorption (therefore Vd and $t_{1/2}$ must be the same - this is not the case in pregnancy).
3. X-ray following barium meal.
4. Scintigraphic techniques measuring uptake of radioactive substances.
5. Ultrasound, which is technically difficult.
6. Impedance; potential tomography; a full stomach has a lower impedance.

● ●

11. WHAT ARE THE POTENTIAL PROBLEMS ASSOCIATED WITH DELAYED GASTRIC EMPTYING AND WHAT ARE THE CAUSES ?

➡ **The problems are aspiration of stomach contents, alteration in the absorption characteristics of oral drugs, and nausea and vomiting. ITU patients typically have delayed gastric emptying.**

Causes:

1. Physiological

- Food and increased osmotic load (jejunal receptors delay emptying to allow controlled release)
- Posture (especially in neonates)
- Anxiety ('state' more important than 'trait')
- Age (some delay in liquid emptying in the elderly)

2. Pathological

- GI obstruction
- Acute gastroparesis
  - Migraine
  - Acute gastro-enteritis
  - Hypercalcaemia
  - Electrolyte imbalance
  - Diabetes Mellitus
  - Raised intracranial pressure
- Muscular disorders
- Anorexia nervosa
- Acute renal failure
- Crohn's disease
- Myxoedema

3. Pharmacological

- Opioids including partial opiate agonists such as meptazinol, nalbuphine, buprenorphine and nefopam
- Epidural opioids
- Anticholinergics
- Atropine
- Tricyclic antidepressants
- Ganglion blockers
- Aluminium and Magnesium hydroxides
- Sympathomimetic drugs
- Salbutamol
- Isoprenaline
- Dopamine
- Alcohol

4. Other Factors
(action less clear cut)

- Pregnancy; no consistent effect BUT does delay paracetamol absorption due to increases in volume of distribution
- Obesity: Solid emptying is **increased, but** liquid emptying is **normal;** the residual volume of gastric secretions is **higher**

• •

6 QUESTIONS ON RENAL PHYSIOLOGY

1. CAN YOU DESCRIBE THE COUNTERCURRENT MECHANISM OF THE KIDNEY?

➡ **You must know this.**

➡ **A countercurrent fluid mechanism is one in which fluid flows through a long U-tube with the two limbs of the U tube lying in close proximity so that exchange of constituents may take place between the two arms.**

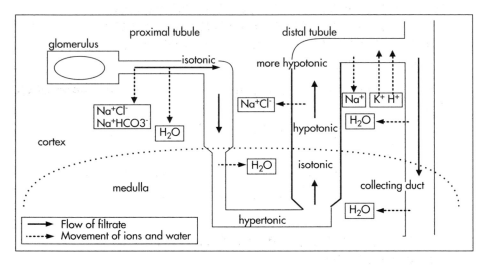

In the loop of Henle, osmolality at the tip is 1200 mosm/l in the lumen and in the interstitium.

The Key is that the ascending limb (the thick portion, which is known as the diluting segment) is impervious to Na^+ and Cl^- ions and has a powerful Na^+ pump moving Na^+ and Cl^- ions into the interstitium. This maintains the composition of the interstitium of the renal medulla at high osmolality.

The purpose is that extremely dilute urine is generated at the distal tubule, which then passes through the highly concentrated milieu of the medulla. The barrier between the two is formed by the collecting duct, whose normally impervious wall can be made permeable to water by the action of ADH. The osmolality of the urine can be adjusted by varying the permeability of the collecting duct to water.

●●●●●●●●●●●●●●●●●●●●●●●●●●●●●●

2. WHAT ARE THE PRESSURES WITHIN THE GLOMERULUS?

➡ **Hydrostatic pressure is higher in glomerular capillary beds than in other organs.**

High capillary pressure is maintained by balance between afferent (precapillary) and efferent (postcapillary) arterioles. Hydrostatic pressure is normally maintained at about 90 mmHg.

Against this is:

- 25 mmHg plasma oncotic pressure
- 15 mmHg Bowman's capsule hydrostatic pressure.

Therefore filtration pressure is about 50 mmHg. This is consistent with:

- The filtration function of the kidney.
- Oliguria being an early feature as arterial pressure falls.

....

3. WHAT HAPPENS TO THE CONCENTRATION OF SODIUM, GLUCOSE AND INULIN AS THE FILTRATE PASSES DOWN THE PROXIMAL CONVOLUTED TUBULE?

➡ **2/3 of water reabsorption takes place in the proximal convoluted tubule (PCT).**

- Inulin is filtered but not reabsorbed, therefore its concentration rises.
- Glucose concentration is zero.
- Sodium concentration is unchanged; water is reabsorbed with sodium.

....

4. HOW IS GLOMERULAR FILTRATION RATE CONTROLLED?

➡ **Glomerular filtration is the volume of fluid filtered from glomerular capillaries into Bowman's capsule per unit time. It is 180L/day in the adult.**

Glomerular filtration rate (GFR) is proportional to glomerular capillary pressure. This in turn depends on:

1. Local autoregulation, mediated by renal sympathetic nerves. Increased sympathetic activity causes increased afferent vasoconstriction, and decreased glomerular pressure.
2. Mean arterial pressure.

....

5. HOW DOES THE KIDNEY EXCRETE H⁺ ION?

➡ **This is all about carbonic anhydrase.**

Control of pH is proportional to $\left\{\begin{array}{l} \text{H}^+ \text{ elimination} \\ \text{HCO}_3^- \text{ reabsorption} \end{array}\right.$

- The intracellular buffers are phosphates and proteins (especially Hb)
- The extracellular buffer is principally bicarbonate (and some proteins)
- The urinary buffers are HPO_4^{2-} and NH_3, and a very little bicarbonate

A diagram may provide an opportunity to explain and for further discussion: start by drawing the renal cell, and the CO_2 and H_2O within it:

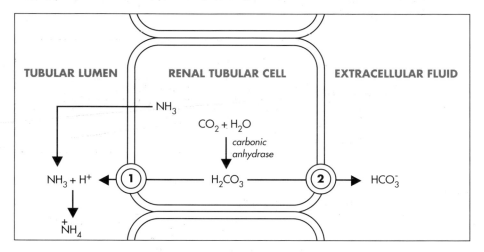

The separate parts of the tubular system are driven by two distinct processes as the transport at **1** and **2** above differ:

A. Early tubular segments (proximal tubule, thick segment of the ascending limb of the loop of Henle and distal tubule):

- At **1**: H^+ is secreted by Na^+/H^+ countertransport (a process driven by the lower intracellular concentration of sodium).
- At **2**: The sodium is then transported out of the cell to the extracellular space by Na^+/K^+-ATPase, and HCO_3^- passes out to balance the electrical effect of the extra sodium pumped out.

B. Late tubular segments (late distal tubules then on through the remainder of the system to the renal pelvis):

- At **1**: H^+ is secreted by primary active transport utilising a specific transport protein H^+-transporting ATPase.
- At **2**: The HCO_3^- is exchanged for a chloride ion that passes out to the tubule with the hydrogen ion and so ensures electrical neutrality.

• •

7 QUESTIONS IN METABOLIC PHYSIOLOGY AND BIOCHEMISTRY

1. WHAT IS MEANT BY NEGATIVE FEEDBACK?

➡ **Negative feedback involves a closed loop and is a homeostatic feature of many biological systems. The hypothalamic-pituitary axis includes many examples of this.**

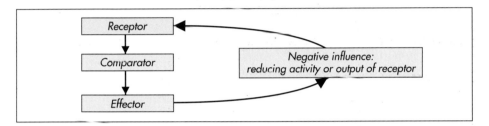

Gain is $\dfrac{\text{amount of correction}}{\text{amount of abnormality remaining}}$

So, increasing the gain gives more correction for the same amount of abnormality.

••••••••••••••••••••••••••••••

2. WHAT IS POSITIVE FEEDBACK?

➡ **This is the opposite of negative feedback, in other words where activity of the effector in a system causes increased (rather than decreased) effector activity.**

An example is found at the presynaptic receptor at the neuromuscular junction; the presence of acetylcholine causes more acetylcholine production. Also, luteinising hormone production is governed by positive feedback.

••••••••••••••••••••••••••••••

3. WHAT IS OSMOTIC PRESSURE?

➡ **This is the pressure that would have to be applied to a solution on one side of a membrane to prevent osmotic flow of water across the membrane from a compartment of pure water.**

- Measurement is by depression of freezing point.
- Calculation: see below.

••••••••••••••••••••••••••••••

4. WHAT IS THE DIFFERENCE BETWEEN OSMOLALITY AND OSMOLARITY?

Concentration:

MolaRity is the number of moles per litRe of solution.

MolaLity is the number of moles per kiLogram of solvent.

Osmotic pressure:

Osmolarity expresses mmol per litre of solution.

Oxmolality expresses mmol per kg of solvent.

Measurement:

1. Depression of freezing point: This is the osmotic effect exerted by sum of all dissolved molecules and ions across a membrane permeable only to water.
2. Calculated:

Total = 2 [$Na^+ + K^+$] + [urea] + [glucose]

N.B.

1. All units are mmol/l
2. The factor of 2 for Na^+ and K^+ allows for equal quantities of associated anions and assumes complete ionisation.
3. Normal serum osmolarity is 290 mmol/l.

Significance:

1. Direct measurement by depression of freezing point indicates osmolaLity.
2. Calculation indicates osmolaRity.
3. Urine contains no protein, whereas plasma contains about 70 g/l of protein. This means that the total volume (water + protein) is about 6% greater than that of the solvent (the water alone). Measured osmolaLity will be greater than calculated osmolaRity.
4. In reality, there is little difference between osmolaRity and osmolaLity other than when there is extreme hyperlipidaemia or hyperproteinaemia.
5. Comparison of plasma and urine must be done in terms of osmolaLity of both, in other words, by direct measurement.
6. Total osmotic pressure of plasma is 7 atmospheres.

••••••••••••••••••••••••••••••

5. WHAT ARE THE ACTIONS OF INSULIN?

➡ **Insulin is the main anabolic hormone, and its action is opposed by all stress hormones.**

1. Activation of glucose uptake.
2. Concurrent uptake of $[K^+]$.
3. Glycogen synthesis.
4. Increased lipogenesis.
5. Inhibition of gluconeogenesis.
6. Inhibition of glycogenolysis.
7. Inhibition of ketogenesis.
8. Inhibition of lipolysis.
9. Enhancement of protein synthesis from amino acids.

••••••••••••••••••••••••••••••••

6. WHERE IS IRON PRESENT IN THE BODY, AND HOW IS IT ABSORBED?

➡ **Iron is present in the body as follows:**

- 50% in haemoglobin, Hb
- 25% in ferritin
- 25% elsewhere

The functions are:

1. In globin, within *haemoglobin*, as O_2 binding site for *transport*.
2. In globin, within *myoglobin*, as O_2 binding site for *collection and storage*.

Only 10% of total iron ingested is absorbed. Active transport transfers iron from the gut to ferritin within the intestinal cells and then to the liver. Ferritin effectively regulates the uptake of iron; the more body iron, the more intestinal iron, and the less iron absorbed.

- Ferritin (mostly hepatic) is a storage protein iron complex.
- Transferrin is a plasma protein (transport).

Most of the intestinal cell ferritin is lost when the cell reaches the top of the villus and drops off.

Conclusion

The affinity of ferritin for iron is reduced when iron is scarce – by an unknown mechanism – allowing more iron to enter circulation and bind transferrin.

••••••••••••••••••••••••••••••••

7. WHAT IS NORMAL EXTRA CELLULAR FLUID VOLUME AND HOW IS IT MEASURED?

➡ **Extracellular fluid (ECF) is 20% of body weight. ECF is one third of total body water.**

ECF is distributed:
- Intravascularly: 4L.
- Interstitially: 10L.

Measurement is difficult because few substances mix readily. Lymph cannot be measured separately. Substances cross the blood brain barrier slowly and don't equilibrate well.

Measurement is also difficult because of the existence of transcellular fluids:
- Glandular secretions.
- CSF.
- Aqueous humour.

The method commonly described is of radioactive Inulin, which has a molecular weight of 5200; using a ^{14}C substitution and dilution technique. (Inulin is also used in measurement of GFR) Cl^- and Br^- labelling doesn't work because these molecules are intracellular.

$$\text{Volume} = \frac{\text{quantity injected}}{\text{concentration observed}}$$

•••••••••••••••••••••••••••••••

8. WHAT IS THE ANION GAP?

➡ **The anion gap has been used to calculate plasma acidity**

$$= ([Na^+]+[K^+]) - ([Cl^-]+[HCO_3^-]); \text{ normal} = 10\text{-}15 \text{ mmol/l.}$$

The anion gap is increased by:
- Increased serum lactate - but lactate can be directly measured now, so the anion gap has become a less frequently used measurement.
- Ketoacidosis.
- Increased foreign anions, salicylates for example.
- Hypocalcaemia.
- Hypokalaemia.
- Hypomagnesaemia.

The anion gap is decreased by:
- Hypoalbuminaemia.
- Increased plasma cations.

•••••••••••••••••••••••••••••••

9. WHAT IS AN EXPONENTIAL FUNCTION?

➡ **One where rate of change of V is proportional to V.**

Examples:
- The rate of flow of liquid from a large container through a narrow hole is proportional to the volume of liquid remaining.
- The rate of metabolism of a drug is proportional to the amount of drug remaining (this is first order kinetics).

The time constant τ relates to the progress of an exponential function had the **initial** rate of change continued.

After   1 τ, 37% of original value remains;

        2 τ, 13.5% of original value remains;

        3 τ, 5% of original value remains.

······························

10. HOW IS BODY WATER DISTRIBUTED?

➡ **Body water is 60% of body weight.**

TOTAL 42L   - Intracellular 24L

              - Extracellular   Plasma 4L

                           Interstitial 8L

                           Dense connective tissue ⎫
                                             ⎬ 6L
                           Bone   ⎭

In:			**Out:**		
	Fluid	2500		Urine	1500
	Food	750		Skin	600
	Metabolic	350		Resp	400
		2600		Stool	100
					2600

Total Secretions: (most of which are reabsorbed)

Saliva	1500
Gastric	2500
Bile	1000
Pancreas	700
Small gut	3000
	$\simeq 9000$

$\simeq 9000$ ml/day; implications for fistulae are obvious.

······························

11. WHAT ARE THE FUNCTIONS OF CALCIUM IN THE BODY?

➡ **Apart from the 99% of the total which is in bone, calcium is a predominantly extracellular ion; when it is present in the intracellular compartment, it exerts profound effects and is a component of many second-messenger systems.**

1. Bone salt: Ca^{++}: PO_4^{2-} 2:1, as $Ca_{10}(PO_4)_6(OH)_2$.
2. Glycogen breakdown requires transient Ca^{++} release to activate phosphorylase kinase.
3. Muscle contraction: Depolarisation causes Ca^{++} release from sarcoplasmic reticulum, affecting the TpC component of troponin, which in turn elicits a tropomyosin-actin conformational change; this causes a contraction.
4. Release of acetylcholine depends on presence of Ca^{++} in the extracellular fluid.
5. Calcium is a neurotransmitter in the generation of the visual impulse, by closure of Na^+ gates.
6. Clotting: Calcium is factor IV in the intrinsic and extrinsic pathways.
7. Vasoconstriction: Calcium is the biochemical antagonist of K^+.
8. The plateau of the cardiac action potential depends on slow Ca^{++} channel activity.
9. It is a positive inotrope.

••••••••••••••••••••••••••••••

12. WHICH AMINO ACIDS ARE ESSENTIAL?

➡ **"Little most – valuable – player"**

Leucine

Isoleucine

Threonine

Tryptophan

Lysine

Methionine

Valine

Phenylalanine; hence tyrosine is not essential unless phenylalanine is absent.

••••••••••••••••••••••••••••••

13. HOW IS PHOSPHATE PRESENT IN THE BODY?

1. Phosphate is present in association with calcium, as the anion.

2. It is present as a buffer in glomerular filtrate to allow excretion of H^+ and generation of HCO_3^-.

3. It is a component of high energy phosphate bonds; adenosine monophosphate, (AMP), adenosine diphosphate (ADP), and adenosine triphosphate (ATP). Insulin facilitates cellular PO_4^- uptake.

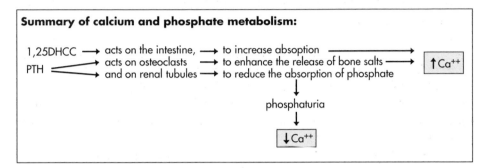

Calcitonin opposes these actions

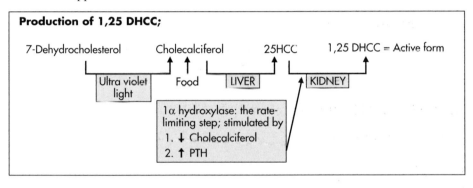

....

14. WHAT COMPONENTS ARE IN TOTAL PARENTERAL NUTRITION (TPN)?

➡ **The indications for TPN may be absolute, for example ileus or extensive bowel resection; or relative, for example cachexia.**

- WATER:

1 -10 kg body weight: 100 ml/kg

10 -20 kg body weight: further 50 ml/kg

Beyond 20th kg body weight: 10 ml/kg

- POTASSIUM: 1.5 mmol/kg/day (1g = 13.5 mmol)
- SODIUM: 1.0 mmol/kg/day
- ENERGY: in kCal = water requirement in ml; 25 - 35 non-protein kCal/kg/day
- NITROGEN: 0.2 - 0.4 g N_2/kg/day (monitor urea)
- MAGNESIUM: 1 mmol/g N_2
- PHOSPHORUS: 0.5 - 0.75 mmol/kg/day
- WATER SOLUBLE VITAMINS
- TRACE ELEMENTS: Zn^+ 100 mmol, Cu^{++} 20 pmol, Mn 5 µmol, Se 0.4 µmol.
- ESSENTIAL FATTY ACIDS.

Maximal rate of glucose infusion = 6.0 mg/kg/min.

Calorie: Nitrogen ratio (KCal:g)

- Malnourished, otherwise well = 200:1
- Catabolic, sick = 80:1

••••••••••••••••••••••••••••••

15. WHAT SUBSTANCES CROSS THE PLACENTA?

> ➡ **The placenta is a single cell - thick barrier; it secretes Renin; the oxyhaemoglobin dissociation curve favours the fetus; maternal hyperventilation causes hypoxia in the fetus.**

Drugs.

Lipophilic neutral drugs, such as volatile anaesthetic agents and propofol, are readily transferred. Weak electrolytes, acids (thiopentone) and bases (local anaesthetics (LA) and opiates), are transferred in the unionised state. Thus bases will accumulate in the fetal circulation, especially if the fetus is acidotic. Polarised molecules (neuromuscular blockers (NMB)) are hardly transferred at all.

Fetal–maternal ratio (FMR).

At equilibrium, a drug will be distributed between the fetus and the mother, depending on the drug's chemical properties. The FMR describes this. An ideal drug would have a very low FMR, in other words, hardly appear in the fetal circulation following administration to the mother. Bupivacaine thus has a FMR of 0.3, lignocaine 0.5, but diazepam has a FMR of 2.0, and so accumulates in the fetus. Pethidine has an initial FMR of 1.0, but this rises with time. Pethidine and its metabolites may be detected in the fetal circulation 7 days postnatally after maternal administration.

So:

- Low-molecular weight, lipid-soluble drugs cross most easily.
- Local anaesthetics cross but not in relevant quantities.
- Non-depolarising relaxants are highly ionised and so don't cross.

•••••••••••••••••••••••••••••••

16. CAN YOU COMPARE THE NERNST AND GOLDMAN EQUATIONS?

➡ **Nernst describes the electric potential necessary to balance a given ionic concentration gradient across a membrane so that the net passive flux of the ion is zero.**

This is analogous to osmotic pressure - the effort required to stop movement.

$$E = \frac{RT}{zF} \log_e \left[\frac{C_o}{C_i} \right]$$

E   = equilibrium potential of the ion in question

C_o, C_i = extra and intracellular concentrations

z   = valance of ion in question

R   = gas constant 8314.9 J/kg.mol.K

T   = absolute temp in Kelvin

F   = Faraday constant = quantity of electricity in 1 mole elections

         = 96, 484 6 c/mol

For Potassium:

$$E = \frac{8314 \times 310}{1 \times 96,484} \times \log_e \frac{4}{140}$$

$$E = 26.7 \times \log_e 0.028$$

So, the larger the extracellular [K^+], the larger the potential difference.

➡ Goldman takes account of Na, Cl and other ions.

$$V_m = \frac{RT}{F} \log_e \frac{P_K \times K_o + P_{Na} \times Na_o + P_{Cl} \times Cl_i}{P_K \times K_i + P_{Na} \times Na_i + P_{Cl} \times Cl_o}$$

P = membrane permeabilities - which can alter, so turning the Goldman equation into the Nernst equation for that particular ion.

•••••••••••••••••••••••••••••••

17. WHAT IS THE CHEMISTRY OF PYLORIC STENOSIS IN THE NEONATE?

➡ **The key is the fact that in normality secretion of HCl into the gastric lumen is balanced by generation of equivalent amounts of HCO_3^- by the parietal cells.**

Normally this is followed by secretion of HCO_3^- into the duodenum. If vomiting occurs with free communication stomach to duodenum, HCO_3^- is vomited out along with HCl. If however there is obstruction between stomach and duodenum, there is no loss of HCO_3^-, Na^+, and K^+.

So; $\uparrow$pH (metabolic alkalosis) $= 6.1 + \log \dfrac{[HCO_3^-]\uparrow}{0.2 \times PCO_2}$

Correction depends on urinary bicarbonate. Hypoventilation does not occur as a compensation to any extent.

However there is loss of Cl^-, and less Cl^- available in the renal tubules to be resorbed along with Na^+;

➡ **Sodium control is paramount. Na^+/K^+ exchange takes over from Cl^- and Na^+ absorption, so Na^+ is absorbed in exchange for K^+; K^+ is therefore lost in both urine and vomit.**

Worse still with K^+ really low, and Cl^- already low, Na^+ must still be conserved; but now not by exchange with K^+ but with H^+; this produces an acid urine, while there is a metabolic alkalosis.

Pyloric stenosis is all about

1. Obstruction between stomach and duodenum and mismatched loss of electrolyte and buffer from those two sites.
2. The overriding need to conserve Na^+ in the kidneys which prevents correction of the problem.

The Paradox of Pyloric stenosis is that while there is vomiting loss of K^+ and H^+, these ions are still excreted in the urine in order to maintain Na^+.

The result is

1. Hypochloraemic alkalosis.
2. Hypokalaemia.
3. Haemoconcentration.

• •

18. HOW ARE CYTOKINES IMPLICATED IN THE DEVELOPMENT OF SEPSIS?

Cytokines are low molecular weight proteins that act as local factors in inflammatory and immune responses. They have a short half-life but are extremely potent, interacting with receptors on membrane surfaces. The actions of cytokines are exceedingly complex and there is considerable overlapping of actions, as well as positive feedback and amplification (as with the complement cascade). They are believed to be the final pathway for the organ and cell damage that is the result of sepsis. The important cytokines are interleukin-1 (IL-1), interleukin-6 (IL-6) and tumour necrosis factor (TNF), and their actions are summarised in the following table:

Cytokine	Source	Activating factors	Effects
IL-1	Vascular endothelium Vascular smooth muscle Macrophages	Tissue injury Exotoxin Endotoxin TNF Complement	Reduced systematic vascular resistance Fever Amplification of TNF effects
IL-6	Vascular endothelium	TNF C5a complement factor	Synthesis of acute phase proteins Fever
TNF	Vascular endothelium Vascular smooth muscle Macrophage	Tissue injury Exotoxin Endotoxin TNF Complement	Reduce systemic vascular resistance by enhanced vasodilatation and reduced vasoconstriction Lactic acidosis Hypoglycaemia Expression of adhesion molecules on vascular endothelium Margination and adherence of neutrophils, monocytes and lymphocytes Activation of neutrophils Increased vascular permeability Self-amplification Release of IL-1 and IL-6 Release of catecholamines, glucagon, cortisol, PAF, arachadonic acid derivatives, interferons

8 QUESTIONS ON ANAESTHETIC DRUGS

1. CAN YOU COMPARE DIAZEPAM, CHLORAL AND TRIMEPRAZINE AS PREMEDICANTS?

	Oral preparation	Antisialogogue	Sedation	Amnesia	Antiemetic	Extrapyramical side effects	Postoperative Pallor	Gastric irritation
Diazepam (Benzodiazepine)	✓	✗	✓	✓	✗	✗	✗	✗
Chloral (Dichloral-phenazone)	✓	✗	✓	✓	✗	✗	✗	✓
Trimeprazine (Phenothiazine)	✓	✓	✓	✓	✓	✓	✓	✗

....

2. WHAT ADVANTAGES DOES HYOSCINE HAVE OVER ATROPINE?

➡ **This is a very common question.**

- Hyoscine has a shorter duration of action.
- Hyoscine produces less tachycardia.
- Hyoscine produces fewer arrthythmias.
- Hyoscine is a more powerful antisialogogue.
- Hyoscine crosses the blood–brain barrier and so produces more central sedative effects.

But:
- It is not such a good bronchodilator.
- It causes more marked effects on the eye.
- Hyoscine causes confusion in elderly and so should not be used in the over-65 age group.

....

3. WHAT ARE THE TOXIC EFFECTS OF LOCAL ANAESTHETICS?

➡ **These can be due to overdose, as part of the therapeutic effect, or due to the addition of a vasoconstrictor or other additive; anaphylaxis is very rare.**

Due to overdose:

a. Central nervous system: Esters (procaine and cocaine) cause central nervous system depression, while amides (the rest) cause central nervous system depression then fits, in other words, there is a biphasic response.

b. Cardiovascular system: Hypotension and brady-arrhythmias.

c. The total spinal.

As part of therapeutic effect:

a. Respiratory depression in intercostal block.

b. Autonomic blockade (spinals).

Vasoconstrictor addition:

a. Digital extremities and gangrene.

b. Vasopressors.may cause a hypertensive crisis if used where psychiatric drugs such as uptake-1 inhibitors are present.

Specific effects:

a. Type I hypersensitivity (Ester group, seen with cocaine).

b. Prilocaine can cause methaemoglobinaemia, for which methylene blue is the specific antidote.

Safe doses :

- Bupivacaine 2 mg/kg
- Lignocaine 3 mg/kg (without adrenaline), 7mg/kg (with adrenaline).
- Prilocaine 5 mg/kg

....

4. COMPARE BUPIVACAINE AND LIGNOCAINE.

➡ **They are both are amide local anaesthetics but have different properties in terms of potency, duration of action and physical characteristics.**

	Bupivicaine	**Lignocaine**
Potency	4	1
Duration	4	1
Safe max. dose (mg/kg)	2	3
PKa	8.1	7.7
Partition coefficient	28	3
Protein bound	95%	64%

....

5.   WHAT DRUGS ARE USED FOR SPINALS?

➡ **All have been used but in contemporary practice lignocaine may be used, although it is more common to use bupivacaine 0.5% with dextrose 5% to achieve hyperbaricity.**

This question would lead on to discussion of aspects of administration, as follows:
- Position: May influence spread of local anaesthetic.
- Spinal curvature: This has an influence on pooling of local anaesthetic, and if this occurs in the caudal curve it may be responsible for the cauda equina syndrome which has been observed in conjunction with the use of spinal micro-catheters. These have fallen out of favour in the United States where their licence had been withdrawn by the FDA.
- Barbotage: This practice may accelerate the spread and onset of a block.
- Interspace: This clearly dictates the level at which the onset of block will be observed, but the eventual extent of the block will not be affected by the level at which it is inserted.
- Volume: Using a larger volume of a lower concentration may elicit a faster onset although this is disputed by many.
- Specific gravity: The baricity will cause the agent to descend and pool in a curve, as discussed above.
- Dose: The total amount of agent dictates the eventual extent of the block. For example, 2 ml of 0.5% bupivacaine will create a block from T4 to S5 in an obstetric patient. This equates to 10 mg of bupivacaine. 10 ml of 0.1% bupivacaine, which is also 10 mg, will also create a block from the upper thoracic region to S5.
- Fixation: Local anaesthetic is fixed to tissue after 20 minutes and is unlikely to extend beyond the established block after this time.

6.   CAN YOU COMPARE CENTRAL NERVOUS SYSTEM TOXICITY OF AMIDE AND ESTER LOCAL ANAESTHETICS?

➡ **Procaine is an ester, as is amethocaine and cocaine; lignocaine and most others are amides.**

The signs of local anaesthetic toxicity in the nervous system are alterations of conscious level and circumoral tingling. Amides cause initial central nervous system depression, which is then followed by convulsions. Ester local anaesthetics produce no biphasic pattern, just central nervous system depression.

7. WHAT IS MAC?

➡ **Minimum alveolar concentration (MAC) of inhalational anaesthetic agent at sea level, in 100% oxygen, at which 50% of unpremedicated experimental animals will fail to respond to a standard midline incision. This is MAC 50; if considering the concentration which will achieve absence of movement in 90% of patients, then this will be MAC 90. The accepted standard is MAC 50.**

The term minimum is used because it is a threshold level; and it is described as alveolar because it applies at equilibrium.

· ·

8. WHAT FACTORS MODIFY MINIMUM ALVEOLAR CONCENTRATION (MAC)?

➡ **Minimum Alveolar Concentration is the amount of the agent delivered in oxygen at room temperature at sea level which will keep 50% of unpremedicated experimental animals still at skin incision.**

It is reduced by:

1. Age (by 10% per decade).
2. Premedication.
3. Opioids.
4. Hypovolaemia.
5. Reduced temperature.
6. Other drugs: for example, clonidine, dexmedetomidine.
6. Disease: hypothyroidism.

· ·

9. WHAT PRESERVATIVES ARE IN A BOTTLE OF LOCAL ANAESTHETIC?

➡ **This question is about spinals and epidurals, which must be performed using agents free of preservatives, because to do so carries the risk of causing arachnoiditis.**

- Single dose ampoules with no adrenaline have no preservative or additive, unless they are hyperbaric preparations, which contain glucose 80 mg/ml.
- Single dose ampoules with adrenaline contain sodium metabisulphite, unless for dental use.
- Multiple dose containers contain methyl parahydroxybenozate 1 mg/ml.

· ·

10. WHAT IS IN THE THIOPENTONE AMPOULE?

The drug is prepared as a sodium salt. It is a 2.5% powder of 5 Ethyl, 5' methylbutyl thiobarbituric acid; pH is 10.5. All salts of weak acids are alkaline in solution.

The preparation also contains 6 parts per 100 of Na_2CO_3 which produces OH^- ions in solution thus preventing precipitation of free acid form of drug. The powder is presented in an atmosphere of nitrogen in order to prevent oxidation in the bottle.

•••••••••••••••••••••••••••••••

11. DOES ENFLURANE HAVE ANY ADVANTAGES OVER HALOTHANE?

- Hepatitis is less frequently observed with enflurane.
- There is less reduction in stroke volume.
- There are fewer arrhythmias.
- Enflurane is a more active muscle relaxant.
- Enflurane is half as potent, and has a more rapid onset of action.

•••••••••••••••••••••••••••••••

12. WHAT FACTORS MODIFY THIOPENTONE DOSAGE?

➡ **"Modify" implies both enhancement and reduction of effects.**

An enhanced effect is seen in:

- The elderly.
- Malnutrition (because of reduced protein binding).
- The debilitated.
- Hypovolaemia.
- Premedicated patients.
- Hyperventilation, which is also a phenomenon of displacement from protein binding.

Reduced effects are seen in:

- Enzyme induction (Hepatic P450 mixed function oxidase).

•••••••••••••••••••••••••••••••

13. WHAT IS THE SIGNIFICANCE OF THE OIL-GAS PARTITION COEFFICIENT?

➡ **It is an index of potency and is inversely related to MAC. This lends itself to a diagram.**

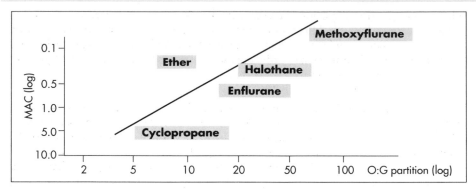

This supports the Meyer-Overton hypothesis of the mechanism of action of anaesthetics, namely that the action is related to the lipid solubility of the agent and takes place at the level of the central nervous system cell membrane. If the Meyer-Overton hypothesis were correct, then the product of MAC and the oil:gas partition coefficient would be a single constant. However the MAC-O:G product produced by the newer agents (sevoflurane, desflurane and isoflurane) is approximately 100 and that of the older agents (e.g. enflurane and halothane) is approximately 200, perhaps suggesting two different sites of action or mechanisms.

The multi-site expansion hypothesis suggests that the sites at which anaesthetics operate have finite size and limited occupancy. When considering volatile agents, MAC is additive, but although opiates reduce MAC they do not do so in a predictable, additive fashion, which suggests that they are not having the effect at the same site as the anaesthetic agent. There is also evidence that anaesthetic agents work at synaptic level, possibly at the thalamic level of the central nervous system.

·····························

14. HOW IS N$_2$O MANUFACTURED?

➡ **By heating Ammonium Nitrate to 245°C**

$$NH_4\,NO_3 \rightarrow N_2O + 2H_2O$$

The end product may contain impurities:

- Ammonia
- Nitric Acid
} On cooling these combine to form $NH_4\,NO_3$

- Nitrogen
- Nitric oxide (NO)
- Nitrogen dioxide (NO$_2$)
} Aluminium dryers will remove these; N_2 evaporates off by distillation

·····························

15. WHAT IS THE SIGNIFICANCE OF THE BLOOD:GAS PARTITION COEFFICIENT?

➡ **There has always been confusion among candidates between the oil:gas, and the blood:gas, partition coefficients.**

The blood:gas (B:G) partition coefficient describes the partition of a volatile anaesthetic agent between blood and gas at equilibrium. Poorly soluble agents have a low B:G coefficient, whereas highly soluble agents will have a high coefficient. Desflurane and cyclopropane have B:G coefficients around 0.4, whereas diethyl ether and methoxyflurane have B:G coefficients of 12.

There is a paradox in the relationship between B:G solubility and rapidity of action. A highly soluble agent will enter the blood avidly, but exert a low partial pressure. The effects on the central nervous system are related to the partial pressure of the agent, not to the absolute amount present, so a soluble agent will have a slow onset of action. A poorly soluble agent by contrast will exert a rapid effect. Thus cyclopropane was a very effective agent for the gaseous induction of anaesthesia, although desflurane, which has a similar B:G coefficient, is limited in its effectiveness for gaseous induction by the irritation it causes in the respiratory tract. Speed of onset also relates to speed of emergence, and desflurane is associated with a rapid recovery whereas methoxyflurane has a very slow pattern of recovery. Methoxyflurane is no longer used in human practice because of concerns about nephrotoxicity, however it remains a useful agent in veterinary practice because of the one property that made it popular in human practice; it is a potent analgesic.

••••••••••••••••••••••••••••••

16. WHAT IS THE NATURE OF ENTONOX?

- $N_2O : O_2$, 50 : 50
- Stored at 137 Bar in cylinder sizes G(3200L) and J(6400L)
- Provided in a blue cylinder, with blue and white quartered shoulders.
- Separates at -7° which is the 'pseudo-critical' temperature: the liquid contains N_2O with very little O_2 dissolved in it.

The existence of Entonox relies on the Poynting effect. The mixed gases do not behave as might be predicted from the characteristics of their components, but rather the two gases appear to dissolve into one another. The mixture is less likely to separate into two phases, under the influence of pressure, than N_2O alone. Thus the mixture is able to remain gaseous at higher pressures and at lower temperatures than N_2O.

••••••••••••••••••••••••••••••

17. WHAT CAUSES HALOTHANE HEPATITIS?

➡ **Halothane is not a classic toxin, because it does not meet the three criteria for a toxin.**

1. Observed dose-effect relationship.
2. Validity in different animal species.
3. Recognised mode of action.

Halothane undergoes oxidative and reductive metabolism to produce trifluroacetic acid, chloride, bromide and fluoride. There are two degrees of hepatic damage observed:

1. Reversible damage, associated with mild elevation in hepatic transaminases; this may be sub-clinical.

2. Fulminant necrosis, which is associated with an antibody-antigen reaction. Halothane behaves as a hapten, binding covalently with hepatic proteins, inducing formation of antibodies. This is supposed to be associated with serial and repeated anaesthetics with halothane, and is seen at an incidence of between 1:82,000 and 1:200,000 in children, although the incidence of unexplained jaundice in adults following halothane anaesthesia is higher, at between 1:2,500 and 1:36,000. The diagnosis of halothane-induced liver damage can only be made after exclusion of all other causes of liver damage.

••••••••••••••••••••••••••••••

18. WHAT ARE THE DEGRADATION PRODUCTS OF SEVOFLURANE?

➡ **Sevoflurane is widely used in Japan but has only recently entered clinical practice in the UK because of fears about degradation products.**

Sevoflurane is broken down by soda lime to $CF_2=C(CF_3)-O-CH_2F$, which is known as compound A. The rate of generation of this compound is not accelerated by soda lime being hotter than usual as first thought, and there remains doubt about the toxicity of this compound. Sevoflurane has been used for many years in Japan including use in circles. It has a rapid onset, like desflurane, but is more pleasant to breathe, has a lower MAC and is more easily administered. It therefore shows great promise and its introduction into clinical practice has been eagerly awaited by many.

••••••••••••••••••••••••••••••

19. WHAT IS THE SECOND GAS EFFECT?

➡ **This is to do with the much smaller solubility of N_2O than N_2, and the influence of this on P_AO_2 and the alveolar concentration of a volatile anaesthetic agent.**

The concentration effect is the effect of rapid extraction from the alveolus of a gas introduced at high concentration, such as nitrous oxide. Because the blood : gas solubility of nitrous is very low, the initial uptake of the nitrous oxide from the alveolus will be high. The alveolar partial pressures of other simultaneously administered gases (such as volatile anaesthetic agents) will therefore be increased. The second gas effect is effectively a consequence of this, as the F_A/F_I (alveolar fraction to inspired fraction) ratio of the concurrently-administered volatile agent will equilibrate faster than it would in the absence of the nitrous oxide. This means that induction of anaesthesia will be more rapid.

The second gas effect has another consequence. In addition to accelerating induction, the effect may retard recovery by causing "diffusion hypoxia". During emergence from anaesthesia, when air is replacing anaesthetic gas, the nitrous oxide will diffuse from the blood to the alveolus faster than it is replaced in the blood by nitrogen from room air, because of the difference in their solubilities. The ratio of the solubility of nitrous oxide to nitrogen is 1:35. Therefore the alveolar concentration of nitrous oxide rises, and if the inspired gas is room air, then the partial pressure of oxygen in the alveolus will be reduced below that of room air by the nitrous oxide entering the alveolus faster than the nitrogen is leaving the alveolus. This is why oxygen is routinely administered to patients emerging from anaesthesia; they would otherwise become hypoxic.

· ·

20. WHY SHOULD VAPORISERS BE EMPTIED FROM TIME TO TIME?

1. In case of inadvertent 'downstream' contamination.
2. To allow servicing.
3. To remove non-volatile additives such as waxoline blue, which was put in trichloroethylene as a colouring agent, and thymol which is in halothane as a stabiliser. Thymol, if allowed to accumulate, impairs evaporation and causes sticking of working parts. You may have noticed sticky trails of thymol on the anaesthetic machine beneath the halothane vaporiser.

· ·

21. WHAT WOULD BE THE IDEAL VOLATILE ANAESTHETIC AGENT?

➡ **The ideal inhalational agent will have physical characteristics, pharmaco-kinetic characteristics, and pharmacodynamic characteristics.**

Physical:
- Stable in light, heat, metal, soda lime.
- No preservatives.
- Long shelf life.
- Not flammable or explosive.
- Non-irritant.
- Atmospherically friendly.
- Cheap.

Pharmacokinetic:
- High oil:gas coefficient, low minimum alveolar concentration (MAC).
- Low blood:gas coefficient, fast effects.
- Not metabolised.

Pharmacodynamic:
- Non-toxic, even in chronic, low dose.
- Absence of, or at least predictable, cardiovascular and respiratory effects.
- Analgesic.
- Readily reversible anaesthetic effects.
- Not epileptogenic.
- No interactions.
- No effects on the gravid uterus.

➡ **You need to memorise all the indices and coefficients of volatile anaesthetic agents before entering the exam hall.**

	Minimum alveolar concentration	Boiling point	Saturated vapour coefficient	Blood: Gas partition coefficient	Oil: Gas partition coefficient	Molecular weight
Halothane	0.7	50	33%	2.3	224	197
Enflurane	1.7	56	24%	1.8	98.5	184
Isoflurane	1.17	49	33%	1.4	99	184
Sevoflurane	1.9	55	24%	0.6	53	200
Desflurane	6.0	23	88%	0.4	20	168

••••••••••••••••••••••••••••••••

22. DRAW THE INSPIRED CONCENTRATION AGAINST THE ALVEOLAR CONCENTRATION FOR A VOLATILE ANAESTHETIC AGENT.

➡ **This is all to do with the blood: gas partition coefficient.**

Poorly soluble volatile agents have a small blood:gas partition coefficient, so alveolar concentration rises rapidly towards inspired concentration, a large gradient exists and onset of anaesthesia is rapid .

N_2O	0.5
Trilene	9.0, - so no good for induction
Cyclopropane	0.4
Halothane	2.3
Enflurane	1.8
Isoflurane	1.4
Sevoflurane	0.6
Desflurane	0.4, fastest of all

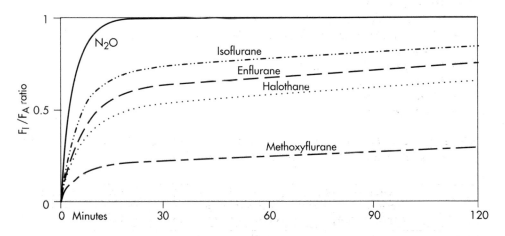

The F_A/F_I ratio rises faster (and therefore induction is faster) in *low* cardiac output and *high* minute ventilation.

••••••••••••••••••••••••••••••••

23. WHAT DOES SATURATED VAPOUR PRESSURE SAY ABOUT AN INHALATIONAL AGENT?

➡ **Saturated vapour pressure (SVP) is inversely related to boiling point and is the concentration of vapour over a liquid when saturation is achieved. It can be a percentage of atmospheric pressure, or an absolute figure if the units are known.**

SVP dictates the calibration of the vaporiser, e.g. halothane and isoflurane both boil at around 50°C and have an SVP of 33%, and so both can be used in the same vaporiser (although not at the same time). Desflurane on the other hand boils at 23°C and has an SVP of 88%.

Vapour pressure is affected by temperature but is independent of barometric pressure, however when the SVP of a liquid reaches barometric pressure the liquid is "boiling" and the temperature is the "boiling point" of the liquid.

••••••••••••••••••••••••••••••••

24. WHO DISCOVERED THE COMMONLY USED ANAESTHETIC VAPOURS?

➡ **Volatile anaesthetic technology was a by-product of the atomic bomb project, as uranium hexafluoride was found to be an essential intermediary in the formation of enriched uranium-235.**

Halothane was synthesised by Suckling in the ICI laboratory in Cheshire in 1951, and introduced into clinical practice in 1956. Between 1959 and 1966, Terrell and others at Ohio Medical (which is now part of BOC) synthesised over 700 agents in an attempt to identify the ideal agent. Of this series, number 347 was enflurane and number 469 was isoflurane. Enflurane was used clinically for the first time in 1971. The introduction of isoflurane into practice was delayed by concerns about toxicity (and in particular carcinogenesis) and so it was not until 1980 that it entered clinical use in America, and 1985 in the United Kingdom. Desflurane was number 653, halogenated entirely with fluorine, requiring a potentially explosive step in the manufacturing process. Desflurane has only recently become available in the United Kingdom.

••••••••••••••••••••••••••••••••

25. WHY DOES ALFENTANIL START TO WORK SO MUCH FASTER THAN FENTANYL, AND WHY IS ITS DURATION OF ACTION SO MUCH SHORTER ?

➡ **This concerns the pharmacokinetic differences between the two drugs. The relevant data is shown in the following tables:**

Drug	Distribution $t_{1/2}$ (min)	Terminal $t_{1/2}$ (min)	Initial volume of distribution (l/kg)	Volume of distribution (l/kg)	Clearance (ml/min)
Fentanyl	13	190	0.85	4.0	1500
Alfentanil	11.6	100	0.16	0.53	240

Drug	Plasma protein binding (% bound)	pKa	% Ionised at pH 7.4
Fentanyl	83	8.4	91
Alfentanil	90	6.5	11

It can be seen that the terminal half-life of alfentanil is half that of fentanyl, but that the clearance of alfentanil is much smaller. Therefore the shorter terminal half-life is due to the smaller volume of distribution of alfentanil - fentanyl is highly lipid soluble and extensively taken up by fat and muscle (this is the main reason for its short duration of action when compared with morphine which has a similar terminal half-life).

As alfentanil is poorly lipid soluble it has a much smaller initial volume of distribution and as it is a weak base (pKa 6.5) the unbound drug is largely (nearly 90%) unionised, so it is allowed rapid access to the brain as it is the unionised molecules that cross the blood-brain barrier. Thus when equipotent doses are given the initial plasma concentration of alfentanil is at least 100-times higher than that of fentanyl and there is very little time lag for an effect to be seen in the brain (using spectral edge analysis) whereas with fentanyl a three minute time lag is seen before peak effect occurs. Thus the half-time for plasma/brain equilibration is 1.1 minutes for alfentanil and 6.4 minutes for fentanyl.

....

26. WHAT IS THE CSM?

➡ **The CSM is the Committee for safety of medicines.**

Adverse reactions should be reported to The Committee on Safety of Medicines, London SW8 5BR using the Yellow Card scheme. With newer drugs, (denoted with an inverted traingle in data sheets and in the British National Formulary) all reactions should be reported. With established drugs, serious suspected reactions should be notified.

....

27. WHAT DO THE LUNGS DO TO SUFENTANIL?

➡ **The lungs are capable of uptake, storage, release and metabolism of many substances.**

Sufentanil is a basic, lipophilic agent which undergoes significant first-pass retention in the lungs. The significance of this is that the binding sites may be saturable, and that in the presence of another, similar, compound there may be displacement of sufentanil from the binding sites with increased quantities of the drug released into the circulation. There are at least two binding sites, however, and saturation does not occur with sufentanil in clinically-used concentrations.

·······························

28. WHY HAS FENTANYL A SHORTER DURATION THAN MORPHINE?

➡ **The shorter duration of action of fentanyl is related entirely to redistribution; clearance is actually slower than that of Morphine. 10% is excreted unchanged.**

However because it is a weak base, it is initially eliminated from plasma to stomach. Subsequent reabsorption from the small intestine causes a secondary rise in plasma levels, and can be responsible for respiratory depression in recovery.

·······························

29. WHAT MAY BE USED TO TREAT METABOLIC ACIDOSIS?

➡ **In adults, the commonly-used agent is sodium bicarbonate 8.4%, which contains 1 mmol bicarbonate per ml.**

Requirement = Base excess x kg body weight x 0.3. It is usual to administer half this amount and re-measure the base excess before administering further bicarbonate.

However there are advantages of hyperventilation over the administration of bicarbonate, especially if the acidosis is of a respiratory nature. Bicarbonate becomes carbon dioxide by the effect of carbonic anhydrase, which merely provides a carbon dioxide load which has then to be eliminated. Bicarbonate may also cause a paradoxical intracellular acidosis, it presents a sodium load, and is hyperosmolar. For these reasons it should be administered with care. However it has a definite place in lactic acidosis, which may be divided into two categories; where there is accompanying hypoxia (type A) and where there is no hypoxia (type B). Bicarbonate is of use in type B lactic acidosis.

·······························

30. DISCUSS THE ANAESTHETIC DOSAGE IN HYPOTHYROIDISM.

➡ **First, delay elective surgery pending adequate correction, unless the patient is presenting for cardiac surgery.**

The disease is characterised by the following implications for anaesthesia:
- Obesity, slow mental and physical function.
- Drug distribution is delayed.
- Drug metabolism is retarded.
- There may be concurrent adrenal insufficiency.

So:
- In the emergency situation, it is necessary to give T_3, intravenously, in a dose of 10 mg and on a regular basis thereafter.
- Use smaller doses of induction agents and opiates.
- There will be a need to reduce relaxant doses.

••••••••••••••••••••••••••••••

31. WHAT IS AN ALLERGIC REACTION?

➡ **There are four types pertaining to anaesthesia:**

INTOLERANCE: Qualitatively normal, quantitatively abnormal reaction to drug; for example, an exaggerated response to an ACE inhibitor.

IDIOSYNCRACY: Qualitatively abnormal, but not immunologically-mediated, response to drug, e.g. gum hyperplasia with anticonvulsants.

ANAPHYLAXIS: IgE-mast cell histamine release reaction, type I hyper-sensitivity.

ANAPHYLACTOID: Direct histamine release from mast cells and macrophages, may be complement-activated; e.g. X-ray contrast medium or althesin.

The manifestations are cutaneous (flushing and urticaria), cardiovascular (hypotension and cardiac arrest) and pulmonary (bronchospasm). Up to 300 patients die in the UK every year from allergic reactions directly associated with anaesthesia.

••••••••••••••••••••••••••••••

32. HOW DO YOU MANAGE AN ALLERGIC REACTION?

➡ **You must have an immediate action drill ready for this type of question.**

1. Stop administration of suspected agent. *CALL FOR HELP !*

2. 100% O_2.

3. Cardiac massage if no pulse.

4. Adrenaline 0.5 - 1.0 ml of 1:10,000.

5. Nebulised bronchodilators.

6. Chlorpheniramine 10 mg.

7. Steroids.

8. Plasma expansion 70 ml/kg, via large bore intravenous cannula.

9. Aminophylline 250 mg slowly.

Aminophylline has considerable problems associated with its use. It cannot be given through a central line because of its arrhythmogenicity, which will be enhanced in the presence of hypoxia and hypercarbia. The dose must be given over 20 minutes, and it may not be possible to exclude the possibility that the patient has not taken aminophylline in the recent past.

·····························

33. WHAT IS MENDELSON'S SYNDROME?

➡ **Curtis Mendelson was an obstetrician in New York, and published his classic paper in 1945.**

He actually described two distinct aspiration syndromes.

1. Solids, producing laryngeal or bronchial obstruction.

2. Liquids, causing an asthmatic - like syndrome with cyanosis, tachycardia and dyspnoea. He identified hydrochloric acid as being responsible.

"The acid produces a bronchiolar spasm, and a peribronchiolar congestive and exudative reaction interfering with normal intrapulmonary circulation to the extent that cardiac failure may develop", but with **NO** mediastinal shift and **NO** massive atalectasis.

The experimental animal was the rabbit and survival endpoint was to be "able to carry on rabbit activities uninhibited".

·····························

34. HOW DO YOU INVESTIGATE AN ALLERGIC REACTION?

➡ **This is about histamine and tryptase.**

➡ **The diagnosis of a reaction must then be followed by the identification of the causative agent.**

Histamine is pathognemonic of the mast cell degranulation which characterises an anaphylatic reaction. However detection of histamine is difficult as the plasma half-life is only 2.5 minutes. A metabolite is methylhistamine, which may be detected in the urine. Plasma tryptase is released in parallel to histamine and although its function is unknown it has a long half-life, is stable in EDTA, and readily measured. It is therefore an excellent and specific marker for a drug-induced allergic reaction.

Take blood samples into two EDTA bottles at each of 0,3,6,12 and 24 hours after the event, store at -25°C, and send to The Department of Immunology at The Royal Hallamshire in Sheffield along with immediate and 24-hour urine samples. Telephone them first. It is then possible to evaluate the mechanism of the reaction from the observations, the plasma tryptase levels, and the urinary methylhistamine.

Presentation	Plasma tryptase (µg/m)	Urinary methylhistamine (µg/ml)	Likely mechanism of reaction
Cardiovascular collapse with or without bronchospasm	>20	>30	True type I hypersensitivity
Bronchospasm alone Urticaria in isolation	0	>30	Non-immune reaction, with lungs as target organ. Pulmonary mast cells may behave differently from others.
Hypotension	<20	>30	Complement-mediated, non-immune reaction
Urticaria in isolation	<5	>30	Non-immune; skin as target organ, analogous to pulmonary reaction as above

This allows the diagnosis of allergic reaction to be made. The agent responsible must then be identified. This was previously done by intradermal injection of a diluted sample of the postulated agent, but this resulted in too many false-positives as simple chemical degranulation of exposed mast cells occurs in response to many agents including saline, by this method. Prick testing, performed by a dermatologist under controlled conditions with dilutions of the suspect agents, is a more specific method as the skin scratch brings sensitised lymphocytes to the surface and into contact with the agent. A wheal >1 cm in diameter lasting more than 30 minutes is taken as positive.

....

35. DESCRIBE THE MANAGEMENT OF POISONING

➡ **1. RESUSCITATION.**

2. CANNULATION and samples to lab for immediate paracetamol and salicylates, retain serum for toxicology.

3. HISTORY, from Ambulance crew. Do not trust the patient.

4. EMPTY STOMACH (not in case of paraffin and corrosive ingestion because of the risk of aspiration) and instillation of activated charcoal (even in delayed presentation, as it may interrupt enterohepatic circulation of drugs). Leave a nasogastric tube in place.

5. SECONDARY SURVEY: Chest X-ray, arterial blood gas analysis, urinary catheter.

6. SPECIFIC ANTIDOTES:

β-blockers	atropine, isoprenaline, glucagon
CO	hyperbaric O_2 ($t_{1/2}$ of COHb is 250 min in air, 50 min in 100% O_2, and 22 min at 2.5 bar)
Cyanide	dicobalt edetate 20ml i.v. chelates CN, Na thiosulphate 50ml 25% presents sulphur substrate for enzyme
Opioids	naloxone
Benzodiazepines	flumazenil
Paracetamol	N-acetylcystine
Digoxin	Digoxin-specific Fab antibody fragments (Digibind)
Metals	chelating agents: desferrioxamine, dimercaprol, penicillamine
Organophosphorus	atropine, oximes, pyridostigmine (used for prophylaxis).
Ethylene glycol	ethanol
Sympathomimetics	β-blockers
Phenothiazines	benztropine
Anticholinergics	physostigmine
Oxidising agents	methylene blue

7. SPECIFIC MEASURES: e.g. pacing in tricyclic toxicity.

8. DIURESIS OR DIALYSIS: Keep urinary pH > 6.5 to prevent myoglobin deposition. Mannitol is better than frusemide.

•••••••••••••••••••••••••••••••

36. WHAT ARE THE PROBLEMS IN MANAGEMENT OF SALICYLATE TOXICITY?

1. Salicylates follow mixed kinetics, and so elimination is unpredictable.
2. There will be uncoupling of oxidative phosphorylation, with increased glucose and oxygen usage, which will exacerbate any existing acidosis.
3. Salicylates are highly protein-bound, which reduces the efficacy of attempts to eliminate the drug by dialysis.
4. In adults, it is common to see a respiratory alkalosis, whereas in children a metabolic acidosis is more commonly seen, which is a more serious complication for the same plasma levels.
5. Hyperpyrexia.
6. Hypoglycaemia.

•••••••••••••••••••••••••••••••

9 QUESTIONS ON PHARMACOKINETICS AND PHARMACODYNAMICS

1. WHAT IS MEANT BY HALF-LIFE?

➡ **This is the time taken for the circulating concentration of a drug to fall by 50% from one compartment.**

$$X_t = X_o/2$$

Since $X_t = X_o e^{-kt}$

Where X_t = amount remaining at time t

X_o = amount remaining at time o

k = first order rate constant, units of reciprocal time

Substituting:

$$\frac{X_o}{2} = X_o e^{-kt_{1/2}}$$

Divide by X_o:

$$\frac{1}{2} = e^{-kt_{1/2}}$$

Take logarithms:

$$\ln 2 = kt_{1/2}$$

Rearrange:

$$t_{1/2} = \frac{\ln 2}{k} = \frac{0.693}{k}$$

Half-life is inversely related to the rate of elimination, so that a rapid rate of elimination indicates a short half-life.

The concentration–time graph, which is an exponential curve, becomes linear if the concentration is expressed as a log.

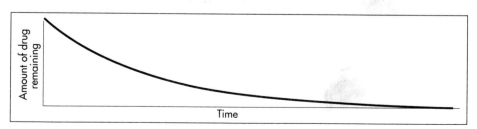

Becomes:

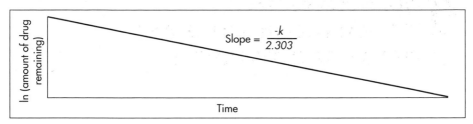

Or, in other words:

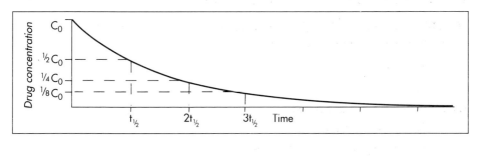

....

2. CAN YOU DEFINE BIOAVAILABILITY?

➡ **Bioavailability refers to the proportion of a drug administered which is then available in the circulation.**

If given by intravenous bolus, there is 100% bioavailability. Oral preparations may undergo first-pass metabolism. Ingestion of the drug and absorption into the portal circulation presents the drug to the liver where it may be extensively metabolised, such that a much diminished amount appears in the systemic circulation. This reduces bioavailability, and the extent to which this happens may differ between preparations of the same drug. Digoxin has been identified as being susceptible to this effect and the variations in bioavailability between different preparations of the drug are a justification for continuing to prescribe one formulation in preference to any other in a patient whose therapy has been stabilised.

....

3. WHAT IS THE DIFFERENCE BETWEEN ZERO AND FIRST ORDER KINETICS?

➡ **Zero order is where the rate is independent of the amount of drug undergoing the process; first order is where the rate is directly proportional to the amount of drug undergoing the process.**

1. ZERO ORDER

Let X be the amount of drug

$$(1) \qquad \frac{dX}{dt} = -k_o$$

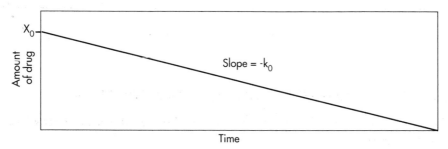

Where $-k_o$ is the zero order rate constant, negative since drug amounts are taken to fall with time; units are mg/min,

e.g. Alcohol

    Phenytoin

    Salicylate

2. FIRST ORDER KINETICS

$$(2) \qquad \frac{dX}{dt} = -kX \qquad \text{compare with (1)}$$

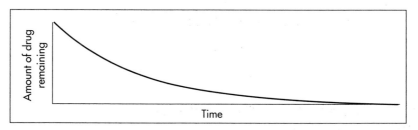

Integrating,

$$(3) \qquad X_t = X_o e^{-kt}$$

Where X_t = amount remaining at time t

        X_o = amount remaining at time o

        k = first order rate constant, units are reciprocal time

Slope is $\dfrac{-k}{2.303}$ since $\log_e 10 = 2.303$

Becomes:

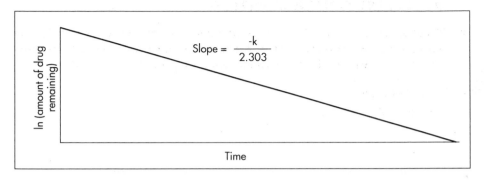

Slope = $\dfrac{-k}{2.303}$

·······························

4. CAN YOU DEFINE VOLUME OF DISTRIBUTION?

➡ **This is the amount of drug administered divided by the concentration of drug observed.**

Take   X   =   Vd x C

At time o, where Vd is the volume of distribution, and rearranging

$$Vd = \frac{X_o}{C_o}$$

In general,   highly protein–bound = small Vd
highly lipid–soluble = large Vd

Also,   Vd < 3L - drug entirely within plasma

Vd > 42L - drug is distributed beyond total body water

·······························

5. WHAT INDICATES THE PRESENCE OF A TRUE RECEPTOR?

• Sensitivity: Receptor-agonist complex produces a predictable result.
• Specificity: Receptor reacts with one type of molecule.
• Saturability: The rate of process is limited by available receptor sites.
• Reversibility: By displacement of agonist or antagonist from the receptor site.

·······························

6. WHAT ARE NON-LINEAR PHARMACOKINETICS?

➡ **Some drugs behave differently at different concentrations.**

E.g. Phenytoin, where the clearance of the drug is dose dependent (first order) until the enzymes involved are saturated, at which point the clearance of the drug becomes constant (zero order) and so the concentration rises much faster as the dosage increases.

D_{max} = the dose at which the curve would become perpendicular
= the asymptote

K_m = C_{ss} at $D_{max}/2$

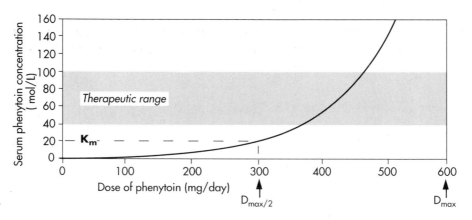

The Michaelis-Menton equation applies:

$$\frac{-dC}{dt} = \frac{D_{max} \times C_{ss}}{K_m + C_{ss}}$$

At low concentrations, i.e. low values of C_{ss}:

$$K_m \gg C_{ss}$$
$$\therefore K_m + C_{ss} \simeq K_m$$

Substituting

$$\frac{-dC}{dt} = \frac{D_{max} \times C_{ss}}{K_m}$$

Simplifying, since D_{max} and K_m are constants for any individual

$$\frac{-dC}{dt} = \text{constant} \times C_{ss}$$

Which is a first order equation.

At high concentrations, and thus high values for C_{ss}

$$C_{ss} \gg K_m$$
$$\therefore K_m + C_{ss} \simeq C_{ss}$$

Substituting

$$\frac{-dC}{dt} = D_{max}$$

Which is a zero-order equation.

Regarding non-linear pharmacokinetics,

1. No constant $t_{1/2}$; it increases with increased dose.
2. Area under the curve (AUC) α dose^2 so a small increase in dose can cause a huge increase in plasma level.

....

7. WHAT IS A HILL PLOT?

➡ **A.V. Hill in 1900 drew PO$_2$ against % oxyhaemoglobin saturation. The Hill plot is also used to mean log dose on x axis against the response, as a proportion, where E is the observed response.**

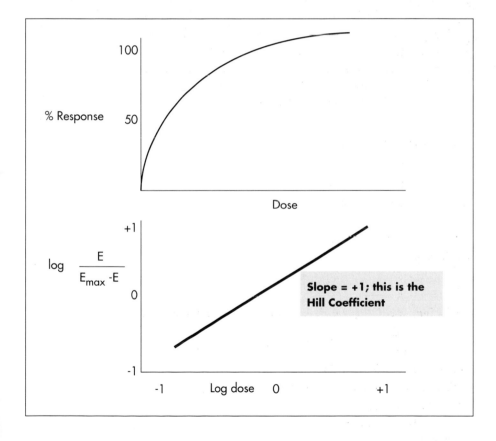

....

8. HOW MAY GENETIC MAKE UP INFLUENCE DRUG ACTION?

1. Fast and slow acetylators: The enzyme N-acetyl tranferase has two phenotypes; this affects the metabolism of, for example, hydralazine.

2. Suxamethonium metabolism: Suxamethonium is metabolised by plasma pseudocholinesterase.

Dibucaine number: this represents % inhibition of enzyme by dibucaine, at 10^{-5} M concentration. Normal is 80% inhibition. A homozygous defect creates an abnormal enzyme with reduced affinity for suxamethonium. This also happens to be resistant to dibucaine inhibition. Fluoride inhibition may also be used to further identify the particular genotype; because there are 4 alleles, there are 10 possible genotypes.

Genotype	Incidence	Response to suxamethonium	Dibucaine number	Flouride number
EuEu	96%	Normal	80	60
EaEa	1:2800	Very prolonged	20	20
EuEa	1:25	Slightly prolonged	40-60	45
EfEf	1:154000	Mod. prolonged	70	30
EsEs	1:100000	Very prolonged	–	–
EuEf	1:200	Slightly prolonged	75	50
EuEs	1:90	Slightly prolonged	80	60
EaEf	1:20000	Mod. prolonged	45	35
EsEa	1:29000	Very prolonged	20	19
EfEs	1:150000	Mod prolonged	60	35

3. G6PD deficiency: This enzyme generates reduced NADPH, which in turn prevents oxidation of cell proteins. The administration of Fava bears and drugs (e.g. sulphonamides, quinine, probenecid) leads to haemolysis.

4. Porphyria. The key to understanding this condition is that it is due to over-production of haem precursors, which are highly toxic, in turn due to the overactivity of the small, readily-induced enzyme δ-aminolaevulinic acid (ALA) synthetase. There is a relative deficiency of an enzyme later on in the synthetic process, thus allowing accumulation of intermediate metabolites. The position of the deficient enzyme predicts the type of precursor to accumulate, and thus, the pattern of the disease, for the smaller intermediates cross the blood brain barrier and cause neuropsychiatric disturbance, while the larger ones cause cutaneous manifestations.

These are uncommon conditions, but the two important conditions are Acute Intermittent Porphyria (AIP) and Variegate Porphyria (VP). Both are inherited in an autosomal dominant form.

Both are precipitated by induction of ALA synthetase by pregnancy, dieting, and drugs of importance such as barbiturates, steroids, sulphonamides and griseofulvin. Management of an attack involves analgesia, carbohydrate loading, β-blockade, fluids and haematin solutions to suppress ALA synthetase activity.

a. Acute Intermittent Porphyria is due to a deficiency of Uroporphyrinogen-1 synthase, allowing accumulation of small metabolites: thus the picture is of abdominal pain, neuropathy, and psychosis. AIP is common in Scandinavia and diagnosis is made by finding ALA in the urine.

b. Variegate Porphyria is due to deficiency of Protoporphyrinogen oxidase, allowing accumulation of large metabolites; cutaneous manifestations of rash and necrosis occur in addition to neurological phenomena, and diagnosis is made by finding porphyrins in the stool.

5. **Malignant Hyperpyrexia.** This is an autosomal dominant condition and is associated with Ca^{++} emergence from the sarcoplasmic reticulum. There is a ratio of 3:1 male:female; and an association with squints and musculoskeletal abnormalities. The incidence is 1:200,000 in the United Kingdom. The diagnosis is based on muscle biopsy, with contracture testing for 0.2 g in halothane 2% and caffeine 2 mmol/l. If positive this is diagnostic and the patient is labelled MH susceptible, or MHS. The term MH equivocal (MHE) is used if one or the other produces a contracture. MH non-susceptible (MHN) is applied if neither produces a contracture, but the test is only 95% sensitive. The condition has a 10% mortality. There is an association with the ryanodine receptor gene, which is located on chromosome 19 q12 - 13.2.

IMMEDIATE ACTION DRILL: CALL FOR HELP

1. Stop trigger agent and stop surgery if possible.
2. Administer 100% O_2.
3. Hyperventilate.
4. Dantrolene (modal effect 2.4 mg/kg, range 1 - 10 mg/kg).
5. Correct acidosis.
6. Correct arrhythmia: anticipate tachycardia and unstable ventricular rhythm.
7. Correct hyperkalaemia, and encourage diuresis; retain urine for myoglobin assay.
8. Cool; use cold fluids, through a blood-warmer containing ice; use a heating system on cold, and apply cold water to the patient.
9. Transfer to ITU and monitor progress of condition by serum CK at 6, 12 and 24 hours.

The morning after diagnosis may be made by assay of myoglobinuria, and a disproportionate rise in plasma CK. Screen proband and family.

•••••••••••••••••••••••••••••••

9. WHAT ARE ACTIVE METABOLITES AND WHICH EXIST FOR MORPHINE AND PETHIDINE?

➡ **An active metabolite has pharmacological action at either the same or a different site as the substance from which it is derived. If the metabolite is more efficacious than the parent compound, the parent can be called a pro-drug.**

Morphine: 70% is metabolised to morphine-3-glucuronide, which has little activity; however, it may be broken down in the gut to release morphine for enterohepatic circulation. Morphine-6-glucuronide, however, has considerable activity at morphine receptors and the distribution of metabolism between the two metabolites may dictate individual response to morphine.

Pethidine: Metabolised to norpethidine, pethidinic acid, and pethidine-N-oxide by phase 1 metabolism in the liver. None have significant effect at the receptor but norpethidine can cause fits and hallucinations.

••••••••••••••••••••••••••••••••

10. WHAT IS AN AGONIST AND AN ANTAGONIST?

An agonist combines with a receptor and achieves a pharmacological response, in other words an agonist has affinity and intrinsic activity.

An antagonist has affinity and has reduced or absent intrinsic activity.

Dose ratio = ratio between doses of agonist required for equivalent response in the presence and absence of the antagonist: a property of a competitive antagonist.

K_a = dissociation constant of receptor - antagonist complex at equilibrium, a measure of the affinity of competitive antagonists for receptors.

••••••••••••••••••••••••••••••••

11. SO WHAT IS pA_2?

➡ **A means of comparing the potency of competitive antagonists.**

It is the negative log of the molar dose of the antagonist in question needed to produce a dose ratio of 2; (where ratio of equivalent doses of agonist in presence of antagonist to absence of antagonist is 2).

For example, for anticholinergics :

- Hyoscine   9.5
- Glycopyrrolate   9.5
- Atropine   9.0
- Largactil   7.5
- Pethidine   5.3

••••••••••••••••••••••••••••••••

12. WHAT IS AFFINITY?

➡ **Affinity is the ability of an agonist to combine with a receptor.**

$$\text{Free Drug + Receptor} \underset{k_2}{\overset{k_1}{\rightleftharpoons}} \text{Drug — Receptor Complex}$$

k_1 = association rate constant

k_2 = dissociation rate constant

At equilibrium, $k_1 = k_2$

So, number of drug molecules (D) combining with receptors is:

$$= \quad k_1 \times [D] \times [R]$$

This must be the same as the number of drug-receptor complexes splitting up:

$$= \quad k_2 \times [DR]$$

But since $k_1 = k_2$

And $\quad k_1 [D] [R] = k_2 [DR]$

$$\frac{k_2}{k_1} = \frac{[D] [R]}{[DR]}$$

$$= k_d$$

Which is the dissociation constant at equilibrium, a measure of AFFINITY.

- If k_d is HIGH there is LOW Affinity.
- If k_d is LOW there is HIGH Affinity.

Similarly k_a is the dissociation constant for antagonist - receptor complex.

....

13. HOW DOES THE LIVER DISPOSE OF DRUGS?

➡ **Aim: To make a lipid soluble drug into a polar, water-soluble product for renal elimination.**

In two stages: Phase I : Non–synthetic, microsomal

Phase II : Synthetic

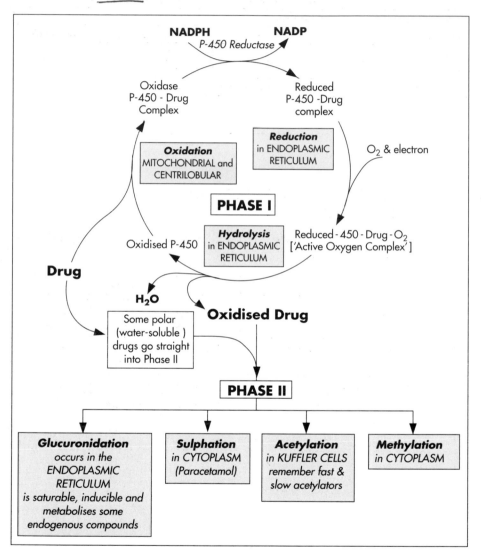

NADPH   NADP
P-450 Reductase

Oxidase
P-450 - Drug
Complex

Reduced
P-450 -Drug
complex

Oxidation
MITOCHONDRIAL and
CENTRILOBULAR

Reduction
in ENDOPLASMIC
RETICULUM

O_2 & electron

PHASE I

Oxidised P-450

Hydrolysis
in ENDOPLASMIC
RETICULUM

Reduced - 450 - Drug - O_2
['Active Oxygen Complex']

Drug

H_2O

Some polar
(water-soluble)
drugs go straight
into Phase II

Oxidised Drug

PHASE II

Glucuronidation
occurs in the
ENDOPLASMIC
RETICULUM
is saturable, inducible and
metabolises some
endogenous compounds

Sulphation
in CYTOPLASM
(Paracetamol)

Acetylation
in KUFFLER CELLS
remember fast &
slow acetylators

Methylation
in CYTOPLASM

. . . .

14. WHERE ELSE MAY DRUGS BE METABOLISED?

➡ Expect the question to lead on to a discussion of the metabolism, or of the drug, that you volunteer as an example.

Location	Mechanism	Examples
Plasma	Pseudocholinesterase	suxamethonium, procaine, propanidid
Neuromuscular junction	Cholinesterase	
Gut wall		lignocaine, chlorpromazine, isoprenaline
Kidney		dopamine
Lung		prilocaine
Hoffman's	Spontaneous degradation	atracurium

. . . .

15. WHAT SECOND-MESSENGERS DO YOU RECOGNISE?

➡ As before, expect a fuller discussion to emerge from the mechanism or example you volunteer.

Mechanism	Example
Ion channel opening/closing	Neuromuscular junction, and the action of noradrenaline on K^+ channels in heart.
Cytoplasmic receptors, increasing mRNA transcription	Thyroid hormones, steroid hormones
Activation of Phospholipase C	Angiotensin II, and the α_2 receptor
Activation of adenylate cyclase (increase or decrease in cAMP)	β_1 receptor, α_2 receptor.
Tyrosine kinase in cytoplasm	Insulin

. . . .

16. HOW IS DIAZEPAM BROKEN DOWN ?

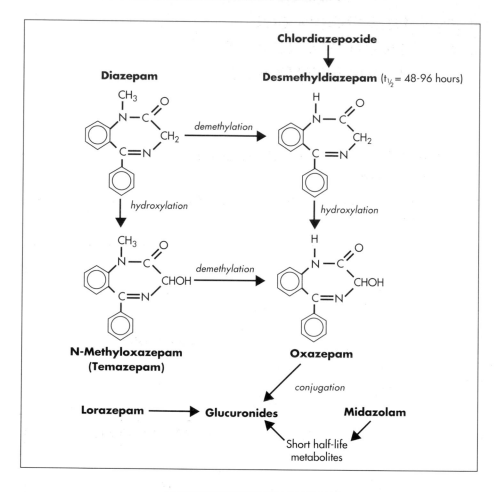

10 QUESTIONS ON CARDIOVASCULAR PHARMACOLOGY

1. HOW IS TYROSINE METABOLISED TO ADRENALINE?

➡ **S**ODOM; **S**ubstitutions = **O**xidation, **D**ecarboxylation, **O**xidation, **M**ethylation

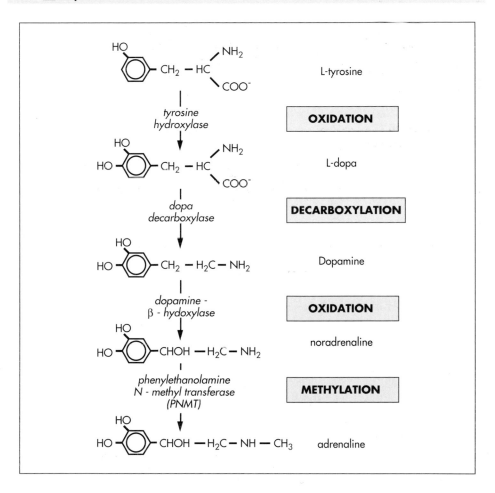

2. CAN YOU CLASSIFY HYPOTENSIVE ANAESTHETIC TECHNIQUES?

➡ **Hypotension may be induced by using anaesthetic drugs which have the side effect of lowering blood pressure, by using specific agents with the intention of causing vasodilation, or by using agents such as labetalol which has several actions.**

As component of drugs employed in anaesthesia:
• Induction: Barbiturates; (Propofol has too short an action in this respect).
• Maintenance: Volatile anaesthetic agents, particularly isoflurane, are potent vasodilators.
• Relaxants: Those releasing histamine, which include curare, gallamine and atracurium.
• Adjuncts: Opiates reduce blood pressure.
• Chlorpromazine, which is an α-antagonist.

Of equal importance in a hypotensive technique, however, is the prevention of a hypertensive response in the first place. This depends on a smooth induction, spraying of the vocal cords with lignocaine, judicious use of opiates and volatiles and the use of a regional technique to induce a sympathetic block.

By vasodilatation and reduction in systemic vascular resistance.

Nitroprusside - affects veins and arteries, and has a half-life $(t_{1/2})$ of a few minutes only.

- The dose is 0.5 - 1.5 µg/kg/min rising to 8.0 µg/kg/min.
- It must be protected from light.
- Nitroprusside is metabolised to cyanide.

Hydrallazine - this affects arteries more than veins.

- The dose is 10-20 mg intravenously, and it has a $t_{1/2}$ of 4 hours.
- There is a bimodal pattern of metabolism, due to fast and slow acetylation, and it may induce an SLE-type reaction.

Labetalol.

Presentation: Clear solution in ampoules of 100 mg in 20 mls as HCl.

Class: β antagonist action three times as potent as α-antagonist action.

Action: Hypotension, with no intrinsic sympathomimetic activity.

Uses: Controlled hypotension in anaesthesia, and in the management of hypertension.

Dose: 1-4 mg/min i.v. Safe practice is to draw up only as much as is needed-a 20ml syringe full is a dangerous object.

Route of administration: Intravenous.

Onset: Immediate.

Duration of action: 4 hours.

Complications: Irretrievable hypotension and heart failure.

Contraindications: Asthma, cardiac failure, heart block.

Side effects: Rash, postural hypotension.

Elimination: Extensive first pass liver metabolism. The $t_{1/2}$ of labetalol administered by the intravenous route is 4 hours.

Interactions: Action of labetalol is enhanced by other antihypertensives. Cimetidine increases the activity of labetalol.

••••••••••••••••••••••••••••••

3. CAN YOU COMPARE THE CARDIOVASCULAR ACTION OF ISOPRENALINE AND DOPAMINE?

Actions of dopamine:

1. Directly on dopamine receptors; D_1 are mostly depressant, decreasing prolactin secretion and causing nausea; D_2 are mostly excitatory.

2. Indirectly as the substrate for catecholamine synthesis.

Dose	Action on:	Response:
Low doses	D_1 receptors	Renal vasodilation
High doses	β_1-receptor	Positive intropic and chronotropic effects
Very high doses	α -receptor	Tachycardia, and vasoconstriction; in high doses there may even be even renal vasoconstriction

Actions of isoprenaline:
The β_1 and β_2 effects exceed the α effects. There is no D receptor action.

So

- Isoprenaline is a positive chronotrope (dopamine is a positive inotrope and a positive chronotrope).
- Isoprenaline doesn't dilate the renal vasculature; dopamine does, and is used for this purpose. However some authorities claim that dopamine is merely a diuretic.
- Isoprenaline is of more use in bradyarrhthmias, and can be used in complete heart block pending the insertion of a pacemaker.
- Isoprenaline is a bronchodilator, and has been used as such, although newer more specific agents have replaced it for this purpose.
- Isoprenaline dilates the pulmonary artery, and this can be useful in pulmonary hypertension.

•••••••••••••••••••••••••••••••

4. WHAT ACTIONS DO NEUROMUSCULAR BLOCKERS HAVE ON THE CARDIOVASCULAR SYSTEM?

➡ **This is about non–depolarisers as well as suxamethonium.**

Instigation	Intermediary	Observed effect
Suxamethonium, which is formed from 2 acetylcholine molecules	Muscarinic (MII) receptors.	Bradycardia.
Non-depolarising blockers	Histamine release (curare is notable for this)	Reduction in systemic vascular resistance (SVR), a drop in blood pressure and a reflex increase in heart rate.
Muscle relaxation		Diminished cardiac output
Ganglion blockade (at cholinergic receptors)	Reduction in sympathetic tone	Decrease in SVR and BP
Muscarinic MII blockade		Vagolytic action; this is seen with gallamine and pancuronium, because of their tris-quaternary structure.

•••••••••••••••••••••••••••••

5. WHAT IS A SELECTIVE PHOSPHODIESTERASE INHIBITOR?

➡ **There are at least five phosphodiesterase isoenzymes and current research is aimed at inhibiting only those which are of cardiovascular purpose.**

Phosphodiesterase isoenzymes:

I   Associated with calmodulin, and smooth muscle relaxation.

II ?

III Associated with cAMP and cGMP; causing inotropy and vascular and airway smooth muscle relaxation.

IV Associated with cAMP and airway dilation.

V   cGMP; direct platelet aggregation inhibition (diisopyramide)

Lusitropy is the enhancement of the rate of myocardial relaxation.

Methylxanthines (for example, aminophylline) affect all isoenzymes, whereas:

Enoximone

Is a specific phosphodiesterase III inhibitor.

Presentation : Yellow liquid in propyl alcohol for mixture in saline or water.

Class : PDE III inhibitor.

Action : Accumulation of cAMP and protein kinase activity, causing inotropy, vasodilatation, renal dilation and chronotropy.

Uses : Chronic and acute cardiac failure and as a pharmacological bridge to transplantation.

Dose : 0.5 mg/kg loading, then infusion of 20µg/kg/min.

Route : IV only.

Onset of action : Within 15 minutes.

Duration: Half-life is 4 hours.

Complications : Tachyarrhythmias.

Elimination : Hepatic and renal.

Interactions: Enoximone potentiates catecholamines.

•••••••••••••••••••••••••••••

11 QUESTIONS ON MOLECULAR PHARMACOLOGY

1. WHAT IS MEANT BY STRUCTURE-ACTIVITY RELATIONSHIPS?

➡ **This is the relationship between the chemical structure of a drug and its effect. It is the basis of receptor theory described by Langley and Ehrlich.**

For example, barbiturates:

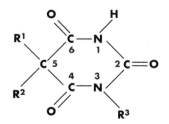

- Larger number of carbon atoms increases potency.
- A phenyl group is anticonvulsant.
- CH_3 at position 1 creates a drug with shorter action and rapid onset.

Sulphur at position 6 makes it a thiobarbiturate, enhancing lipid solubility, speed of action and recovery.

•••••••••••••••••••••••••••••••

2. DESCRIBE THE STRUCTURE OF THE ACETYLCHOLINE RECEPTOR

➡ **This receptor has a pentametric structure consisting of five protein subunits that span the membrane with the channel within them.**

The subunits are as follows:

1 α-subunit (MW 40,000)
- This binds to acetylcholine (Ach).
- The binding of the first Ach molecule improves affinity for the second one.
- The binding of second Ach leads to a configuration change which opens the channel.

2 β-subunit (MW 50,000)

3 γ-subunit (MW 60,000)
- This becomes the ε-subunit in the adult

4 δ-subunit (MW 65,000)

➡ **A drawing is the best way to describe this:**

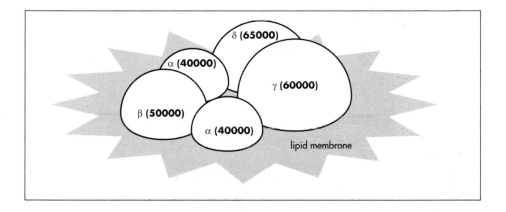

....

3.   HOW IS ACETYLCHOLINE FORMED?

➡ **Acetylcholine is formed at the presynaptic end of cholinergic axons by the transfer of an acetyl group from acetyl CoA to choline.**

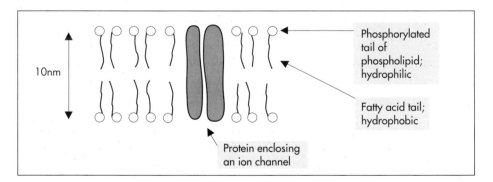

Acetyl CoA is formed from pyruvate + CoA + NAD^+ under aerobic conditions (i.e. from glycolysis via the Krebs cycle) or from Leucine amino acid degradation.

•••••••••••••••••••••••••••••

4.   WHAT IS THE NATURE OF THE CELL MEMBRANE?

➡ **It consists of a lipid bilayer.**

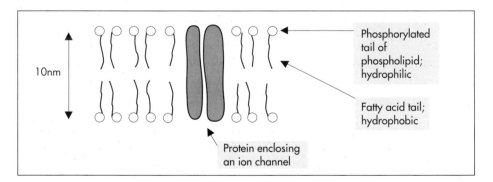

Transfer of substances may occur by means of:

1. Simple diffusion: highly lipid-soluble, non ionised compounds, e.g. alcohols.
2. Non–ionic diffusion "Facilitated diffusion".
3. Active transport: This may be primary (associated with covalent modulation) or secondary (allosteric modulation).

•••••••••••••••••••••••••••••

5. WHAT OPIOID RECEPTORS DO YOU RECOGNISE?

➡ **This is a very popular question.**

Broadly speaking there are three groups, described by Martin according to the ligand associated with each type. Therefore there are μ receptors, for which the ligand is morphine, κ receptors (ketocyclazocine), σ receptors (SKF 10047) and δ receptors, which are named because of being discovered in the mouse vas deferens. The effects at different sites can be tabulated:

	Mu (μ)	**Kappa (κ)**	**Sigma (σ)**
Pupil	Miosis	Miosis	Mydrasis
Respiratory rate	Depression	No change	Stimulation
Heart rate	Bradycardia	No change	Tachycardia
Behaviour	Indifference	Sedation	Delerium
Thermal pain	Analgesia	No effect	No effect
Mechanical pain	Analgesia	Analgesia	Weak analgesia

· ·

6. WHICH AGENTS BIND WHICH OPIOID RECEPTORS?

➡ **Consider natural ligands and then agonists and antagonists in a table:**

	Endogenous ligand	**Selective agonist**	**Selective antagonist**
Mu (μ)	β-endorphins Enkephalins	Morphine Fentanyl	β-funaltrexamine
Kappa (κ)	Dynorphins	U69593, CI-977	Binaltorphamine
Sigma (σ)	Enkephalins	DPEN[2] DPEN[5] enkephalin	Naltrindole

However different opioids may have agonist, partial agonist or antagonist effects at various receptor types:

	Mu (μ)	**Kappa (κ)**	**Delta (δ)**	**Sigma (σ)**
Morphine	Strong agonist	Weak agonist	Weak agonist	No effect
Naloxone	Strong antagonist	Strong antagonist	Strong antagonist	No effect
Fentanyl	Strong agonist	Weak agonist	No effect	No effect
Pentazocine	Partial agonist	Strong agonist	Weak antagonist	Strong agonist
Butorphanol	Partial agonist	Strong agonist	Strong antagonist	Strong agonist
Nalbuphine	Strong agonist	Partial agonist	Weak antagonist	Weak agonist
Buprenorphine	Partial agonist	Strong antagonist	Strong agonist	No effect
Meptazinol	Weak agonist	No effect	Strong agonist	No effect

Antagonist at k receptors

· · · · · · · · · · · · · · · · · · · ·

7. HOW DO BENZODIAZEPINES WORK?

➡ **By facilitation of gamma amino–butyric acid (GABA) neurotransmission.**

Thus:

- Action on limbic system and hypothalamus: Reduces emotional response.
- Action on limbic system and reticular activating system: Diminishes arousal.
- Effect on polysynaptic reflexes in cord: Inhibits synaptic reflexes.

....

8. WHAT IS GABA? HOW DOES IT WORK?

➡ **An inhibitory mediator in the brain and is responsible for presynaptic inhibition. This is to do with transmembrane potentials; a threshold potential must be reached before depolarisation can occur.**

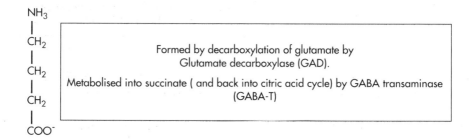

NH_3
|
CH_2
|
CH_2
|
CH_2
|
COO^-

Formed by decarboxylation of glutamate by Glutamate decarboxylase (GAD).

Metabolised into succinate (and back into citric acid cycle) by GABA transaminase (GABA-T)

The excitatory post synaptic potential (EPSP) is proportional to Na^+ entry, opposing the inhibitory post synaptic potential (IPSP) which is proportional to K^+ exit and Cl^- entry.

There are at least two types of GABA receptor;

- $GABA_B$ increases K^+ conductance.
- $GABA_A$ increases Cl^- conductance, and is a true ion channel.

The GABA receptor consists of α, β, γ and δ subunits, analogous to the nicotinic receptor. GABA binds the β subunit and elicits effect. The action is potentiated by benzodiazepines.

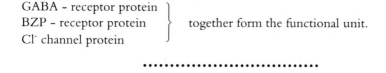

GABA - receptor protein ⎫
BZP - receptor protein ⎬ together form the functional unit.
Cl^- channel protein ⎭

....

9.   WHAT IS THE NMDA RECEPTOR?

➡ **This is the N - Methyl - D - Aspartate receptor, a glutamate receptor in the brain whose action is potentiated by glycine, which is probably essential to its function.**

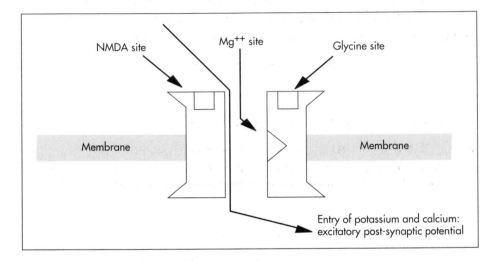

There are at least three types of glutamate receptor; NMDA, Kainate, and quisqualate. Glutamate is the main excitatory neurotransmitter in the brain.

The NMDA receptor embodies a cation channel; this causes increase in the excitatory post-synaptic potential, making the membrane more excitable and more likely to depolarise.

Points:

1. Glycine is required.
2. The channel is blocked by Mg^{++} which only moves when depolarisation is commenced.
3. Phencyclidine and ketamine bind to the channel, like Mg^{++}, decreasing likelihood of depolarisation. This may be the basis of action of ketamine, an NMDA receptor antagonist.
4. There is a high concentration of the receptor in the hippocampus. It is possible that it has a role in memory and learning, by means of "long-term potentiation", which is a long term facilitation of transmission in neural pathways following a period of high-frequency stimulation.
5. It is effectively the antagonist to the GABA receptor.

•••••••••••••••••••••••••••••••

10. WHAT ARE ENKEPHALINS AND ENDORPHINS?

➡ **They are all opioid peptides and are neurotransmitters. They bind to opioid receptors (δ, κ, σ, ϵ, μ).**

Enkephalins:

These are formed from Proenkephalin. they consist of Met-Enkephalin, Leu-Enkephalin, Octapeptide, Nonapeptide. They are found in the substantia gelatinosa and the gastrointestinal tract.

Endorphin:

β-endorphin. It is formed from pro-opiomelanocortin, and is the natural ligand for μ-receptors found throughout the central nervous system, and in the pituitary gland; β-endorphin is an ACTH-precursor fragment.

Dynorphins:

These are formed from prodynorphin, and the group includes:

$\left\{\begin{array}{l}\text{Dynorphin 1-8}\\\text{Dynorphin 1-7}\\\alpha - \text{Neoendorphin}\\\beta - \text{Neoendorphin}\end{array}\right.$

•••••••••••••••••••••••••••••••

11. WHAT ARE STEREO - OR OPTICAL ISOMERS, AND WHAT ANAESTHETIC AGENTS EXHIBIT STEREOISOMERISM ?

➡ **Compounds that show stereoisomerism are those that have an asymmetrical atom.**

Normally in biological systems this is a carbon atom that has four different groups attached to it and so can exist in two forms that have the same molecular formula and geometric structure in two dimensions but have different three-dimensional structure. This is important in physiology because many reactions rely on the approximation of a number of parts of two molecules (e.g. transmitter and receptor), and this is based on their three-dimensional shape so this is stereoselective.

Stereoisomerism is important in anaesthesia because if an anaesthetic agent exhibits stereospecificity it implies that its mode of action involves some form of direct protein interaction, rather than a more general effect by interacting with the lipid membrane surrounding those proteins.

An important example of Stereoisomerism is ketamine. The usual form available is the racemic mixture (an equal mixture of both isomers), and its action and side effects are well known. However the effects of the two isomers are quite different. D-ketamine is four times more potent than L-ketamine. The D form is associated with less agitation and shorter recovery times. At a molecular level the D-isomer has a higher potency on catecholamine high-affinity transport in synaptosomes, and the L-isomer is more potent against serotonin transport. Other agents that have been investigated are etomidate, barbiturates, secondary alcohols and ropivacaine.

Of the inhalational anaesthetic agents halothane isomers have been found to have similar potency, but other agents have not been studied.

L-ketamine   **D-ketamine**

. . . .

12 QUESTIONS ON THE PHARMACOLOGY OF THE NEUROMUSCULAR JUNCTION

1. HOW DOES SUXAMETHONIUM WORK?

➡ **Suxamethonium is a combination of two acetylcholine molecules joined at their acetyl groups, and this is a hint at its action. It is in fact an agonist.**

It acts by mimicking the action of acetylcholine at the post synaptic receptor at the neuromuscular junction. Unlike ACh, it is not metabolised at the neuromuscular junction but in the plasma and so the block persists until the suxamethonium diffuses out of the neuromuscular junction to be metabolised.

....

2. WHAT ARE THE ADVERSE EFFECTS OF SUXAMETHONIUM?

➡ **A very commonly-asked question. Be ready to produce a list, and then discuss one of the adverse effects in detail.**

- Muscle pain: This is extremely common and due to the intense fasciculations seen especially in the young and fit patient.
- Bradycardia: Especially on the second dose. Suxamethonium consists of two acetylcholine molecules.
- Hypotension: This is due to histamine release, muscle relaxation and bradycardia.
- Malignant hyperpyrexia. A whole question in its own right.
- Raised intraocular pressure: This may cause extrusion of eye contents in the penetrating eye injury, although if you talk to those who regularly anaesthetise eye cases, they may tell you this is not the case.
- Increased gastric and intestinal secretion and movement.
- Prolonged paralysis.
- Dual block: This is associated with myasthenia, the Eaton –Lambert syndrome, and concurrent use of anticholinesterases including those present in eye drops.
- Death: Anaphylaxis is relatively common, although death need not be a consequence
- Hyperkalaema: This is a consequence of receptor proliferation, and is seen in burns, tetanus and in upper motor neurone lesions. It is also seen in myotonia dystrophica.

....

3. WHAT IS 'MARGIN OF SAFETY' IN NEUROMUSCULAR TRANSMISSION?

➡ **There is a large safety factor in the transmission process both in acetyl-choline release and in the number of receptors. Both are very much larger than needed to produce the critical degree of endplate potential required to initiate excitation.**

Thus a full sized muscle twitch may be produced in the presence of 75% overall receptor block, whereas a few percent more might result in total absence of contraction; this is the "iceberg" effect.

·····························

4. HOW DO YOU MONITOR NEUROMUSCULAR TRANSMISSION?

➡ **Using a nerve stimulator, which delivers 50 mA for 0.2 - 1.0 msec.**

TWITCH-TETANUS-TWITCH: This distinguishes the *type* of block; four patterns may be observed.

1. Normal; symmetrical twitches followed by sustained tetanic contraction; no post-tetanic facilitation (PTF).
2. Total block; no response.
3. Partial depolarising block; weak but symmetrical twitches, sustained tetanic contraction, no PTF.
4. Partial non-depolarising block; weak twitches, fade on tetanic stimulus, post-tetanic facilitation.

TRAIN OF FOUR: This distinguishes the *degree* of block. It is possible to use the count, or the ratio of force of 4th to 1st twitch (T4:T1).

Count 1,2,3	75% block
Count 1,2	80% block
Count 1	90% block
Count 0	100% block.

POST-TETANIC TWITCH COUNT: This determines the *reversibility* of a block; the device delivers 50 Hz for 5 sec, then 1 Hz, counting detectable twitches. Reversal is possible if count is greater than 10.

DOUBLE BURST: This uses 3 pairs of 50 Hz pulses separated by 0.75 sec. It assesses recovery from block, displaying the T1:T4 ratio.

·····························

5. WHAT IS DESENSITISATION BLOCK?

➡ **This is also known as type II block.**

This is a block elicited by repeated doses of suxamethonium coming to resemble a non-depolarising block. It is said to be due to desensitisation of the neuromuscular junction to suxamethonium, or to inhibition of acetylcholine synthesis. Either way, it is a pre-synaptic effect. It cannot be antagonised by neostigmine.

••••••••••••••••••••••••••••••••

6. HOW DOES NEOSTIGMINE ACT TO REVERSE NEUROMUSCULAR BLOCK?

➡ **The chemical structure of neostigmine resembles that of acetylcholine (ACh), and the acetylcholinesterase enzyme has two binding sites:**

The anionic site binds the cationic part of acetylcholine, and of neostigmine.

The esteratic site binds the terminal carbon atom by forming a covalent bond, serine transferring H^+ to histidine in order for this to take place.

Neostigmine binds to acetylcholinesterase (AChE) and the phenol group is broken away, leaving both binding sites occupied by fragments: the resulting molecule has a $t_{1/2}$ of 40 minutes.

1. Thus ACh metabolism is impaired.
2. ACh accumulates.
3. The non-depolarising, competitive neuromuscular blocker is displaced.
4. Neuromuscular transmission is restored.

••••••••••••••••••••••••••••••••

7. WHAT DRUGS MODIFY THE ACTION OF NON-DEPOLARISING NEURO- MUSCULAR BLOCKERS?

➡ **The actions of non-depolarising blockers are reversed by anti-cholinesterases such as neostigmine; but the effects are enhanced by high dose neostigmine.**

• Aminoglycosides and steroids: These theoretically enhance effects, but this is rarely seen. The effect is related to presynaptic calcium transport.
• Lithium and local anaesthetics: These enhance effects of neuromuscular blockade, by causing a degree of Na channel block.
• Volatile agents: These enhance neuromuscular blockade, by central depression of reflexes and also by direct action at the neuromuscular junction.

Doxapram: This retards the neostigmine-induced antagonism of vecuronium.

••••••••••••••••••••••••••••••••

8. WHAT DO CALCIUM ANTAGONISTS DO AT THE NEUROMUSCULAR JUNCTION?

➡ **Calcium antagonists are synergistic with neuromuscular blocking drugs.**

Patch-clamp recordings suggest that the drug occupies open ion channels and blocks them.

....

9. HOW MAY ANTIBIOTICS INTERFERE WITH NEUROMUSCULAR BLOCK?

➡ **This is a question about aminoglycosides, especially streptomycin and neomycin.**

These antibiotics will enhance neuromuscular blockade, but they are infrequently used in current practice. Historically streptomycin was used for the chemotherapy of tuberculosis, and it prolonged the action of neuromuscular blockade. It was especially difficult to reverse neuromuscular blockade when the agent was present. There was a particular problem with streptomycin when administered intraperitoneally; the effect is thought to be due to impedance of Ca^{++} transport. There may be a neostigmine – resistant block, which in turn can be antagonised by Ca^{++} salts.

....

10. CAN YOU CLASSIFY THE ANTICHOLINESTERASES?

➡ **These act by allowing cumulation of acetylcholine in the in the synaptic gap and so displace the non-depolarising blockers from post-synaptic receptors.**

1. Quaternary ammonium compounds: used clinically

- Neostigmine
- Pyridostigmine
- Physostigmine
- Distigmine
- Edrophonium

2. Organophosphorus compounds: insecticides and chemical weapons

- Dyphlos
- Ecothiopate

....

11. WHAT HAPPENS IF YOU GIVE MIVACURIUM AND SUXAMETHONIUM?

➡ **The dose of any non-depolarising neuromuscular blocker needs to be reduced following the prior administration of suxamethonium. By contrast, the administration of a non-depolarising neuromuscular blocker prior to the use of suxamethonium has an antagonistic effect on the development of a depolarising block.**

The interesting thing about mivacurium, however, is that it is metabolised in the plasma by pseudocholinesterase, at a rate 70% of that of suxamethonium. However it may be that prior administration of suxamethonium does not alter the dose of mivacurium required for adequate relaxation.

Administration of mivacurium prior to suxamethonium, as with other non-depolarising agents, antagonises the development of suxamethonium's depolarising block.

....

13 QUESTIONS ON NON-ANAESTHETIC DRUGS

1. WHAT IS THE MECHANISM OF ACTION OF ANTIBIOTICS?

➡ **These depend on finding a difference between human and bacterial systems; they can be bactericidal or bacteriostatic.**

- Cephalosporins and penicillins inhibit enzymes producing bacterial cell walls.
- Polymyxin and nystatin attach to sterols in fungal cell membranes.
- Sulphonamides act as false substrate by mimicking folate.
- Aminoglycosides and erythromycin inhibit protein synthesis by causing the misreading of RNA.
- Metronidazole inhibits DNA synthesis.

....

2. CAN YOU CLASSIFY THE DIURETICS?

1. Osmotic diuretics – e.g. mannitol: These agents reduce water and electrolyte reabsorption in the proximal convoluted tubule. These are used to reduce intracranial pressure and in certain cases of poisoning. In the management of raised intracranial pressure, mannitol creates an osmotic gradient across the blood–brain barrier and so reduces brain oedema. The diuretic effect follows.

2. Loop diuretics – e.g. frusemide: These inhibit Cl^- (and Na^+) absorption in the thick ascending loop of Henle, and are the most commonly used diuretics.

3. Thiazide diuretics – e.g. chlorothiazide: These inhibit sodium reabsorption in the distal convoluted tubule. These are used in the treatment of hypertension.

4. Carbonic anhydrase inhibitor: Acetazolamide. This is principally used to reduce intraocular pressure rather than as a diuretic.

5. Potassium sparing: Amiloride: This works as do the thiazides, but also inhibits potassium secretion in the distal convoluted tubule as well.

6. Aldosterone antagonists: Spironolactone. The main use of this drug is in the treatment of hyperaldosteronism and other manifestations of chronic renal failure.

....

3. WHAT ARE THE PROBLEMS WITH THIAZIDE DIURETICS?

➡ **These are widely prescribed and it is helpful to be familiar with their problems.**

- Thiazides are diabetogenic.
- They cause an increase in serum urea.
- They are associated with an increase in urate, and the precipitation of gout.
- They cause hypokalaemia, which is of considerable significance for anaesthesia.
- They cause potentiation of action of digoxin and hypotensive agents.
- Thiazides cause lithium retention.

······································

4. HOW IS HEPARIN MANUFACTURED?

➡ **Heparin is a commercial preparation from animal intestinal mucous membranes.**

It is strongly negative charged, and acidic. 1 mg contains 100 units.

······································

5. CAN YOU CLASSIFY THE ANTIEMETICS?

➡ **By site of action.**

Chemoreceptor trigger zone:
- Antidopaminergics: these are the phenothiazines.
- Butyrophenones, for example, droperidol.
- Metoclopramide.
- Antihistamines.

Vomiting Centre:
- Hyoscine.
- Antihistamines.

Gut:
- Drugs which reduce sensitivity: metoclopramide, antacids.
- By $5HT_3$ antagonism: Ondansetron. This has a great future as an effective antiemetic in anaesthetic practice, where its efficacy is proven, but it is rather more expensive than other antiemetics.
- By increasing gastric emptying:
    Metoclopramide.
    Domperidone.

······································

6. WHICH DRUGS MAY BE ADMINISTERED TRANSDERMALLY?

➡ **Transdermal administration has the advantage of avoidance of needles, but the absorption is unpredictable as it depends on local skin perfusion. The absorption will also depend on the formulation, and it may be deliberately delayed, for example with hormone replacement therapy, to provide a continuous low-dose administration.**

1. Nitrates, in the treatment of angina.
2. Steroid hormones in hormone replacement therapy.
3. Hyoscine, as a prophylactic against motion sickness.
4. Fentanyl, as a premedicant for children.

....

7. WHAT ADVERSE EFFECTS DO NON-STEROIDAL ANTI-INFLAMMATORY DRUGS HAVE ON THE KIDNEY?

➡ **All stress hormones, catecholamines and angiotensin II cause vasoconstriction and a reduction in renal plasma flow. The mechanism whereby this is opposed and renal vasodilation occurs is prostaglandin-mediated, by PGI_2; thus in the presence of prostaglandin inhibition, vasoconstriction is unopposed, and if hypovolaemia or hypotension is also present, the kidneys may become ischaemic.**

The following are recognised complications of non-steroidal therapy:

1. Sodium and water retention.
2. Acute renal failure: the commonest complication, especially likely in dehydration, cardiac failure and hypovolaemia.
3. Acute interstitial nephritis.
4. Chronic renal damage.
5. Hyperkalaemic hyporeninaemic hypoaldosteronism.

....

8. WHAT IS THE MECHANISM OF ACTION OF SALICYLATES?

➡ **There are different mechanisms at high and low dosage; this is all about prostaglandin synthesis.**

Eicosanoids are products of arachidonic acid metabolism (Eicosa means 20 carbons)

$$
\left.
\begin{array}{l}
\text{Prostaglandins} \\
\text{Prostacyclins} \\
\text{Thromboxanes} \\
\text{Leukotrienes}
\end{array}
\right\}
\quad
\begin{array}{l}
\text{are locally metabolised, and} \\
\text{rapidly destroyed, therefore these are not hormones.}
\end{array}
$$

These are unsaturated fatty acids with a ring at one end. Prostaglandins A and E are different families; subscript numbers indicate the number of double bonds.

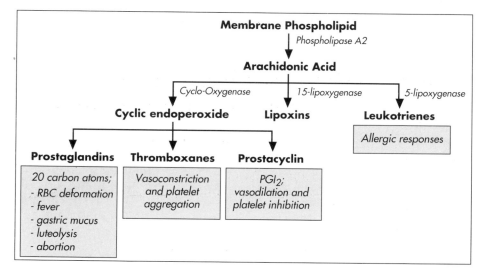

Steroids inhibit arachidonic acid release and so prevent production of all classes of eicosanoids. By contrast, aspirin irreversibly inactivates cyclo-oxygenase by acetylating it. Thus the effects of aspirin last 5-7 days, until more cyclo-oxygenase is synthesised in sufficient quantity. Therefore eicosanoid production is diverted into leukotriene synthesis causing allergic responses in susceptible individuals.

However Aspirin at low dose inhibits platelet cyclo-oxygenase while sparing vessel wall cyclo-oxygenase.

So, thromboxane production is reduced, preventing vasoconstriction and platelet aggregation, while prostacyclin production is spared, allowing vasodilatation and platelet inhibition.

So: finally – actions of aspirin.

1. Cyclo-oxygenase inhibition

   a. Reduced prostaglandin production and reduced pain: Prostaglandins normally sensitise peripheral receptors to bradykinin.

   b. Reduced prostaglandin production and fever: This effect takes place in the hypothalamus.

2. Oxidative phosphorylation uncoupling: This leads to increased oxygen and glucose requirements.

3. Reduced thromboxane production therefore inhibition of platelet adhesion.

4. Urate retention due to diminished tubular secretion (at low dose).

   Urate excretion due to reduced tubular reabsorption (at high dose).

5. Because of increased glucose usage, blood glucose falls.

6. Hyperpyrexia in high dose because of increased cellular usage of oxygen.

··································

9. WHERE DO ANTITHYROTOXIC DRUGS ACT?

1. Carbimazole and thiouracils inhibit iodine incorporation into tyrosine to form thyroxine.

2. Thiouracils and β blockers inhibit the conversion of T_4 to T_3.

3. Iodine inhibits T_4 release from thyroid cells.

4. Radioactive iodine destroys thyroid cells.

5. Potassium perchlorate opposes thyroid stimulating hormone (TSH) in the uptake of iodine by thyroid cells.

··································

14 QUESTIONS ON STATISTICS

1. WHAT STEPS WOULD YOU TAKE TO SET UP A CLINICAL TRIAL?

➡ **This is well described by the appropriate parts of the PROTOCOL. This is the documentation of the intentions and design of a trial, and is the central step in setting up a trial.**

Features of the protocol:

I. Background and general aims:
    a. Why the trial is worthwhile, and how it builds on previous knowledge; a search of the available literature will be required to ascertain the present state of knowledge.

II. Specific objectives:
    a. An exact description of the hypotheses that are being tested. It is always considered statistically more significant to be answering specific questions rather than globally trawling for data then trying to fit questions to the results.

III. Criteria for patient selection:
    a. In order for your sample population to be representative of a larger group, the trial should be focused on patients likely to benefit from the therapy being trialled.
    b. The disease state must be carefully defined to enable the results to be applied to clinical practice in the future.

IV. Criteria for patient exclusion:
    a. Lack of consent should be remembered here.
    b. Other factors that could bias the results of the trial (e.g. other drug therapies) should be entered here to exclude those patients.
    c. Patients who could be harmed by the treatment in question should be excluded.

V. Treatment schedules:
    a. An exact plan of how the treatments will be used should be drawn up.

VI. Evaluation of response:
    a. A plan of what will be measured, how, and by who, both as a baseline and after treatment.

    b. The evaluation should be divided into principle criteria of response, subsidiary criteria and side effects.

    c. What methods are to be used to ensure accuracy and reduce the risk of bias in these results.

VII. Trial design:

    a. Use of a control group.

    b. Randomisation and other methods of treatment allocation.

    c. Blinding.

VIII. Consent and Ethical Committee approval

IX. Required size of study:

    • It is vital to assess the estimated required size from the P value (α-error) and the power (β-error) decided on.

X. Form for data entry:

    • These should be designed now and assessed to remove any ambiguity.

XI. Protocol Deviations:

    • What to do with those patients that do not follow the planned regime.

XII. Plans for statistical analysis:

    • These should be laid down again to ensure that the questions asked are those that are answered not those that happen to be thrown up by the results.

XIII. Administrative responsibility and funding.

........................••••••

2. WHAT ARE α- AND β- ERRORS?

➡ **These are both errors in statistical analysis.**

α-error (or type I error)

This is usually expressed as P = (a number) or P < (a number), and is the probability that a difference will be found despite the two populations being the same (i.e. P = 0.05 means that for twenty trials between identical groups one will show a difference between the groups purely by chance); this is the same as the risk of a **false positive result.**

β-error (or type II error)

This is the probability of not detecting a significant difference between two populations when one does in fact exist; this is the same as the risk of a **false negative result.**

$(1-\beta)$ is known as the power of the study.

........................••••••

3. WHAT ARE MEAN, MODE AND MEDIAN AND HOW ARE THEY RELATED IN A NORMALLY DISTRIBUTED (GAUSSIAN) POPULATION?

➡ **The mean is the 'average' of a population, that is the sum of all the measurements divided by the number in the group.**

➡ **The mode** is the most commonly observed value.

➡ **The median** is that measurement which lies exactly halfway between each end of a range of values ranked in order.

In a normally distributed population they are all at the same point.

In any symmetrically distributed population the mean and the median will be the same, and the difference (mean–median) may be considered to be a rather crude measure of the 'skewness' of the population.

The mode is the highest peak, however the population may be 'mutimodal' by having several peaks, and is commonly 'bimodal' with two peaks – and example of the latter may be a study into the glove sizes of all the people who commonly work in theatre, with peaks at 8 and 6½ for male and female staff respectively.

•••••••••••••••••••••••••••••••

4. WHAT IS FUZZY LOGIC?

In many areas we use "crisp" logic to define precise sets of information; "John is a boy". However defining "tall" as against "short" is not possible in this way. It uses "if" and "then" commands to produce a pathway. For example, to control the speed of a car:

• IF speed is slow THEN accelerate
• IF speed is high THEN decelerate
• IF speed is low AND road is uphill THEN accelerate sharply.

➡ **The application is that it may be used to control certain functions and a recently published example used fuzzy logic to control blood pressure.**

•••••••••••••••••••••••••••••••

APPENDIX 1:

RESPIRATORY GAS CURVES

The Shunt Diagram

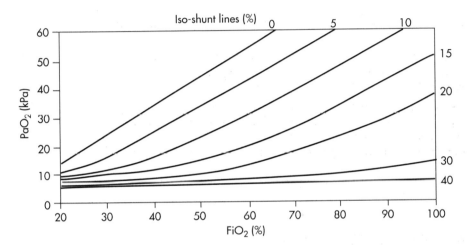

The O$_2$ - CO$_2$ diagram

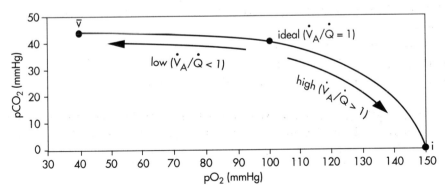

APPENDIX 2:

PHYSIOLOGICAL FORMULAE AND EQUATIONS

Ideal gas equation: $PV = RT$

Where P is pressure, V volume T temperature, and R a constant. At the same temperature, P and V are inversely related; increasing pressure will reduce volume.

Dead space: $V_{D,Phys} = V_{D,Anat} + V_{D,Alv}$

Total dead space ($V_{D,Phys}$) is made up of alveolar dead space (non-ventilated alveoli) and anatomical dead space (conducting airways). Alveolar dead space increases in disease while anatomical dead space increases with age.

Bohr equation:

$$V_{D,Phys} = V_T \times \frac{P_A CO_2 - P_E CO_2}{P_A CO_2}$$

The Bohr equation assumes no CO_2 in inspired gas. The normal physiological (total) dead space, as a proportion of tidal volume, $(V_D/V_T) = 0.3$

To measure $V_{D,Anat}$ use Fowler's method; corresponds to vertical line through phase II of the single breath nitrogen washout. Normal = 150 ml. (see page 40)

Alveolar ventilation equation:

$$V_A = \frac{VCO_2}{P_A CO_2} \times K$$

Where $K = 0.863$, if V_A is body temperature, ambient pressure, and saturated with water vapour (BTPS), and VCO_2 is standard (0°C) temperature and pressure (760 mmHg) and dry (STPD). Essentially, alveolar ventilation is proportional to CO_2 production and inversely proportional to alveolar CO_2.

This is not the same as what follows (although it is a common mistake to confuse the two):

Alveolar gas equation:

$$P_A O_2 = P_I O_2 - \frac{P_A CO_2}{R}$$

The alveolar partial pressure of oxygen is dependant on the inspired fraction and on the amount of CO_2 which is, effectively, displacing the oxygen. This explains the advantage of pre-oxygenation, and explains why desaturation occurs rapidly after apnoea as the CO_2 accumulates in the alveoli unless preoxygenation has been used. It also relates to altitude, and explains the mild hyperventilation seen at altitude – reduction in CO_2 allows more space for oxygen. The equation as written above assumes no CO_2 in inspired gas.

Venous admixture: this is venous blood entering the systemic arterial circulation. Venous admixture is due to frank shunt + the effects of low $\dot{V}/\dot{Q}$. Note that while $\dot{V}/\dot{Q}$ affects O_2 and CO_2, shunt only really affects oxygenation.

Shunt equation:
$$\frac{\dot{Q}s}{\dot{Q}t} = \frac{Cc'O_2 - CaO_2}{Cc'O_2 - C\bar{v}O_2}$$

Normal = 5 ml/100 ml.

Diffusing capacity:

The amount of gas transferred across a membrane is proportional to:

- Area
- Difference in partial pressures
- Constant
- 1/thickness

Diffusing capacity may be measured by the single breath carbon monoxide (CO) technique, where the disappearance of a single breath of CO is measured over a 10 second breath hold. Helium dilution is used to measure total lung volume at the same time.

$$D_L = \frac{\dot{V}CO}{P_ACO} \quad \text{(Normal 25 ml/min/mmHg)}$$

Oxygen flux = cardiac output x oxygen content.

Oxygen content = (1.31 x Hb x Sat/100) + 0.02 PO_2

Henderson–Hasselbalch:
$$pH = pKa + Log_e \left(\frac{[HCO_3^-]}{0.03\ PCO_2} \right)$$

This is used to calculate blood pH, which falls (blood becomes more acid) if the bicarbonate falls or the CO_2 rises.

Laplace's law:
$$P = \frac{4T}{r}$$

Where P is the pressure in a bubble, T is the surface tension and r the radius. A small bubble (or alveolus) will collapse into a large one because it will have a larger pressure within it, due to the action of T in the walls of the alveolus. This does not happen, of course, because of the action of surfactant, which reduces the surface tension .

Pouseille's law:
$$\dot{Q} = \frac{P\pi r^4}{8\eta l}$$

Where $\dot{Q}$ is flow through a tube, P is the pressure difference between the ends, η is the viscosity of the fluid and l the length of the tube. Laminar flow applies. The point is that flow through a tube, vessel or cannula is determined by the driving pressure, the viscosity and the length in a simple manner but is governed by the radius of the tube to the fourth power. So, doubling the radius of a cannula increases flow 16 times.

Reynolds number: $$Re = \frac{2rvd}{\eta}$$

This describes the possibility of turbulent flow, where r is radius, v velocity and d density, with η viscosity as before. If the number exceeds 2000, turbulent flow is likely.

· ·

APPENDIX 3 :

SHORT NOTES ON DRUGS

HOW TO DESCRIBE A DRUG

➡ **A nmemonic: Pretty Cute Anaesthetists Can Undo Dresses Regardless Of Displeasure Clearly Covering Sister's Expression In Theatre:**

- PRESENTATION: Tablets, injection, colour.
- CHEMICAL NATURE: Draw if appropriate, e.g. volatile anaesthetic agents.
- ACTION: At receptor level.
- CLASS: e.g. Vaughan-Williams.
- USES: Stress anaesthetic uses but do not omit those that the rest of the world uses the drug for.
- DOSE: Obvious.
- ROUTE OF ADMINISTRATION: Again, obvious, but don't guess; for example, alfentanil only has a licence for IV use, whereas fentanyl has a licence for IV and IM use.
- ONSET: Rapid, slow or delayed.
- DURATION OF ACTION: Short, medium or long; state the half-life if you know it.
- CONTRAINDICATIONS: Absolute and relative.
- COMPLICATIONS: These are the serious ones like asystole and agranulocytosis, in contrast to:
- SIDE EFFECTS: Which are the less serious ones like nausea and vomiting, but these two (complications and side-effects) do overlap.
- ELIMINATION: Usually hepatic or renal. In general, if a drug is lipid-soluble, it will be absorbed orally, it will cross the blood-brain barrier (BBB) and the placenta, it will be reabsorbed by the kidneys and therefore be eliminated by metabolism and conjugation. If a drug is water-soluble, it will not be absorbed orally, will not cross the BBB or the placenta, and will be filtered by the kidneys.
- INTERACTIONS: With what, and the effect: enhancement, or retardation, of one or the other.
- THE GRAVID UTERUS: See above.

Abbreviations are freely used in this section:

Cl	=	clearance
$t_{1/2}\beta$	=	elimination half-life
MAO	=	mono amine oxidase
COMT	=	catechol O-methyl transferase
MAOI	=	monoamine oxidase inhibitors
Resp	=	respiratory
IV	=	intravenous
IM	=	intramuscular
PO	=	orally
N and V	=	nausea and vomiting
BP	=	blood pressure
HR	=	heart rate
RR	=	respiratory rate
PCA	=	patient-controlled analgesia

•••••••••••••••••••••••••••••

FENTANYL

P : Aqueous solution 100µg in 2mls

C : Narcotic analgesic

A : Agonist at µ opiate receptors

U : Analgesia, premedication, respiratory depression

D : Children, 1-5µg/kg; adults, 50-2000µg

R : Intravenous or intramuscular

O : 1-2 min

D : 30 min (Redistribution more significant than elimination) $t_{1/2}\beta$ 219 minutes

CI : Respiratory failure unless ventilated, MAOI

C : Reduction in blood pressure, heart rate and and respiratory rate, 'Wooden chest'.

S : Nausea and vomiting.

E : 10% eliminated unchanged. Hepatic metabolism. Cl 13 ml/min/kg

I : MAOI; Neuroleptics

GU: Respiratory depression in neonate

•••••••••••••••••••••••••••••

ALFENTANIL

P   : Aqueous solution 1mg in 2mls with NaCl. pKa is 6.5 – all other opiates are basic

C   : Narcotic analgesic

A   : Agonist at μ opiate receptors

U   : Analgesia, respiratory depression

D   : 500 μg, or 30 – 50 μg/kg in IPPV.

R   : IV only; infusion 0.5 – 1.0 μg/kg/min

O   : One arm-brain circulation time

D   : 5-10 minutes $t_{1/2}\beta$ 90 minutes

CI : Resp failure unless ventilated, MAOI

C   : Reduction in blood pressure, heart rate and and respiratory rate, 'Wooden chest'

S   : N and V

E   : Hepatic. Highly lipid soluble Cl 6 ml/min/kg

I   : MAOI, and neuroleptics

GU: Resp depression in neonate

•••••••••••••••••••••••••••••••

PROPOFOL

➡ **2.6 Disopropylphenol.**

OH

$(CH_3)_2HC$ ⬡ $CH(CH_3)_2$

In: Glycerol
   Egg phosphatide
   Sodium hydroxide
   Soybean oil
   Water

P : 1% solution in isotonic medium 20mls

C : 2.6 Disopropylphenol

A : Anaesthesia

C : Anaesthetic induction agent

U : For induction and maintenance of anaesthesia, also sedation in adults

D : 2.5 mg/kg induction, 0.1 mg/kg/min maintenance

R : Intravenous only

O : Within 30 seconds

D : Short, five minutes

CI : Allergy to Propofol

C : Pain on injection, bradycardia, hypotension, apnoea

S : Anaphylaxis; may actually be anti-emetic rather than the opposite; green urine; a report of green hair !

I   : Other anaesthetic agents (enhances), vapours (hypotension, bradycardia)

GU: Not licensed, and not an appropriate induction agent in any case in obstetrics

••••••••••••••••••••••••••••••

CHLORPROMAZINE

P : Tablet or clear solution for injection, as the chloride salt, 1%

C : Phenothiazine

A : See below

U : Major tranquilliser

D : 10-100 mg

R : PO or IM. NOT IV, because of hypotension

O : Rapid

D : 6-8 hours

CI : Hepatic disease, Parkinson's disease, prostatism, glaucoma

C : Cholestasis

S : Extrapyramidal, drowsiness, postural hypotension (α block)

E : Hepatic metabolism and urinary excretion

I : Alcohol, opiates, (enhanced effect); antihypertensives, hypoglycaemics (depressed effect)

GU: Prolongs labour, low Apgar score

Actions:

1. Isolates reticular activating system

2. Antiemetic

3. ↓ Hypothalamic activity

4. Parkinsonian effects

5. ↓ muscle tone

6. Potentiation of analgesics

7. α blockade

8. Muscarinic blockade, like atropine

9. Antihistamine

10. Membrane stabilising activity

11. Anti-5HT activity

•••••••••••••••••••••••••••••••

DROPERIDOL

P : Aqueous solution, 10mg in 2mls, with lactic acid and water

C : Butyrophenone

A : Occupation of GABA receptors

U : Premed/Antiemetic/Neuroleptanalgesia; chemotherapy vomiting; major tranquilliser

D : 0.2 - 0.3 mg/kg

R : IV, IM for premed. oral tablets also available

O : 20 minutes in Rapid IV

D : Up to 48h despite short $t_{\frac{1}{2}}$ (3h)

CI : Comatose states, severe depression

C : ↓ BP, Neuroleptic Malignant syndrome

S : Sedation, Extrapyramidal, oculogyric, NOT anticholinergic

E : Hepatic

I : Opiates, alcohol (enhanced), Protects against catecholamine arrhythmias

GU: Not established

•••••••••••••••••••••••••••••

NALBUPHINE

P : Aqueous solution 20mg in 2ml

C : Narcotic analgesic

A : Affinity for μ receptors with partial agonist activity (some would say antagonist)

U : Premed/operative analgesic/postop inc. PCA

D : 10-20 mg in adult

R : IV, or S/C or IM

O : 10 minutes

D : Prolonged

C : Allergy

C : ↓HR ↓BP

S : Drowsiness

E : Hepatic

I : Alcohol, sedatives

GU: Not known

Nalbuphine is a μ antagonist and a partial κ agonist; buprenorphine is exactly the opposite, a partial μ agonist and a κ antagonist.

•••••••••••••••••••••••••••••

VECURONIUM

P : Freeze dried 10mg with mannitol and preservatives, as vecuronium bromide
C : Non depolarising muscle blocker
A : Competitive antagonist at neuromuscular junction
C : Steroid nucleus
U : Paralysis
D : 80-100 µg/kg initially, then 30-50 µg/kg supplements
R : IV only
O : 120 seconds
D : 25 minutes, longer in children; $t_{1/2}$ = 55 minutes
C : ↓ HR. ? Cumulation in CNS
E : Distribution more than elimination; 30% biliary
I : Enhanced in muscular disease, ↑K+, ↓pH, ↓Ca++, in presence of aminoglycosides, calcium antagonists and volatile anaesthetic agents
GU: None

● ●

ATRACURIUM

P : Clear (faint yellow) 1% solution in 2.5, 5, 25 mls; as besylate; stored at 2 - 8°C
C : Non depolarising muscle blocker
A : Competitive antagonist at neuromuscular junction
C . Racemic mixture of 10 stereoisomers
U : Paralysis
D : 0.3, 0.6 mg/kg, and infusion 0.3-0.6 mg/kg/hour
R : IV only
O : 90 seconds
D : 20 minutes $t_{1/2}$ = 20 minutes
C : Histamine release ↑HR
E : Hoffman degradation to laudanosine
I : Enhanced in muscular disease, ↑K+, ↓pH, ↓Ca++, in presence of aminoglycosides, Calcium antagonists and volatile anaesthetic agents
GU: None

Differences in fade: Vecuronium affects onset more than offset because it has a slower disassociation from presynaptic receptors.

● ●

DOPAMINE

P : Clear solution, some preparations in Dextrose 5% as hydrochloride

C : Catecholamine

A : low dose at D1 receptors, medium dose at β–receptors and high dose at α–receptors

U : renal vasodilatation, then inotropy (more than chronotropy), then vasoconstriction

D : 1-5 μg/kg/min to 5-20 μg/kg/min

R : Intravenous only, via central venous catheter, by infusion

O : Immediate

D : $t_{1/2}$ 2 minutes

CI : Phaeochromocytoma, tachyarrhythmia, MAOI, outflow obstruction

C : Arrhythmia, vasoconstriction

S : N and V, Angina

E : MAO and COMT

I : MAOI

GU: Not teratogenic

••••••••••••••••••••••••••••••

DOBUTAMINE

P : Clear solution, 250 mg ampoule, as hydrochloride, with Na metabisulphite

C : Adrenoceptor agonist

A : Almost solely at β1-receptor; facilitates atrio-ventricular conduction

U : As inotrope in pump failure

D : 2.5-2.0 μg/kg/min

R : IV infusion. Not necessarily by central line

O : Immediate

D : $t_{1/2}$ 2 minutes

C : Arrhythmia

S : N and V, angina

E : MAO and COMT

I : MAOI

GU: Not teratogenic

••••••••••••••••••••••••••••••

ADRENALINE

P : Clear solution as 1:1000 (1g in 1000mls = 1mg/ml)

C : Catecholamine

A : Agonist at $\alpha-$ and $\beta-$receptors

U : Inotrope, chronotrope; resuscitation (vasopressor)

D : Resucitation: 1mg IV, infusion: 0.05 - 1.0 µg/kg/min

R : IV or IM

O : Immediate

D : $t_{1/2}$ = 2 mins

CI : Phaeochromocytoma, arrhythmia, outflow obstruction

C : Vasoconstriction, arrhythmia, ischaemia

S : N and V, tremor, angina

E : MAO and COMT

I : MAOI

....

NORADRENALINE

P : Clear solution 1mg/ml (= 10%, = 1g in 1000 mls)

C : Catecholamine

A : Agonist at $\alpha \gg \beta$ receptors

U : Emergency management of hypotension

D : 0.05 - 1.0 µg/kg/min

R : Intravenous infusion

O : Immediate

D : $t_{1/2}$ 2 min

C : MAOI, Phaeochromocytoma, arrhythmia, outflow obstruction

C : Hypoxia, hypercarbia, with volatile anaesthetic agents there is a tendency to arrhythmia, ↑BP, worsened ischaemia

S : Reflex bradycardia, N and V, angina

E : MAO and COMT

I : MAOI

....

DOPEXAMINE

P : Aqueous solution 1% in 5mls adjusted to pH 2.5, as hydrochloride

C : Adrenergic receptor agonist

A : At β2 and D1 and D2 receptors, also uptake-1 inhibition; No α effect

U : Claimed 100% increase in cardiac output (afterload reduction, by β2 and D1 stimulation), inotrope (β2, U_1 effects), splanchnic perfusion (D1 effect)

D : 0.5-6 µg/kg/min

R : Central vein

O : Immediate

D : $t_{1/2}$ 7 minutes

C : MAOI, outflow obstruction

C : ↓ K^+ ↑Gluc. Tachycardia

S : N and V, Angina

E : MAO and COMT

C : Enhanced effects of adrenaline and noradrenaline

GU: Unknown

....

METARAMINOL

P : Clear solution 1% solution with Na metabisulphite and NaCl

C : Adrenergic receptor agonist

A : Vasopressor far more than inotrope

U : Acute hypotensive crisis secondary to to spinal anaesthesia or shock

D : 0.5 - 5mg bolus; infusion, up to 100mg in 500mls

R : Intravenous

O : One minute

D : 20 minutes to one hour

CI : Ischaemia, arrhythmia

C : Volatile anaesthetic agents

....

GUANETHIDINE (ISMELIN)

P : Clear 1% solution in 1ml with NaCl and Sulphuric acid

C : Sympathetic neurone blocker

A : Depletes and inhibits reformation of noradrenaline at postganglionic endings

U : Hypertensive crisis, and in the management of sympathetic pain. (Guanethidine block)

D : 10-20 mg

R : IV or IM

O : 30 minutes

D : 4-6 hours

C : Phaeochromocytoma, MAOI, renal failure

C : ↑BP initially

S : Dizziness, tremor

E : Partly renal - highly polar drug

I : β-blockers precipitate bradycardia

GU: No study. Ileus in new-born

· ·

PHENTOLAMINE (ROGITINE)

P : Pale yellow 1% solution in 1ml water; as mesylate

C : α1 and α2 blocker

A : Antagonist at a receptor. Also − insulin release

U : Hypertensive crises; failure (↓ afterload); phaeochromocytoma surgery; also, phentolamine test in chronic pain; positive response to IV injection implies longer lasting response to a sympathetic block

D : 5-10 mg IM, 1.5 mg IV

R : IV, IM also PO

O : < 2 minutes

D : $t_{1/2}$ 19 minutes

C : Hypotension

S : Reflex tachycardia, angina, flushing. Tachycardia can obviate usefulness

E : 13% in urine

· ·

NALOXONE

P : Clear sterile solution 400 µg/ml

C : Narcotic antagonist

A : Pure antagonist at all opiate receptors

U : Reversal of opiate side effects and overdose

D : 0–0.4 mg repeated

R : IV (or IM)

O : Immediate

D : $t_{1/2}$ 1 hour – less than the agonist

CI : allergy

C : fits, acute withdrawal syndromes

S : N and V

E : Hepatic

GU: Presumably enters placenta

Structure – activity relationship; all opiate agonists have a methyl group.

•••••••••••••••••••••••••••••••

DOXAPRAM

P : Clear solution 200 mg in 5 mls (also infusion 100 mg/500 ml)

C : Analeptic agent

A : Low dose: peripheral chemoreceptors. High dose: resp. centre

U : Reversal of post-op respiratory depression, and the treatment of acute type II respiratory failure

D : 0.5 – 4.0 mg/kg bolus

R : Intravenous

O : Immediate

D : $t_{1/2}$ 3 hours

CI : Cerebral oedema, coronary artery disease, hyperthyroidism, hypertension

C : Where no CO_2 retention exists

S : Tachycardia, N and V, tremor, convulsions

I : Enhances MAOI, aminophyllines, sympathomimetics, and retards the neostigmine – induced antagonism of vecuronium neuromuscular block

GU: Not recommended

•••••••••••••••••••••••••••••••

DIGOXIN

P : Tablets, 125 µg, 250 µg: injection, clear 0.5 mg in 2 mls

C : Antiarrhythmic

A : Negative chronotrope, positive inotrope, by ATPase inhibition at atrio-ventricular node

C : Steroid nucleus with 5 substitutions

U : Heart failure, supraventricular arrhythmias especially atrial fibrillation and flutter

D : Loading, 0.5 mg, 0.25 mg, oral maintenance: 5 µg/kg o.d.

R : IV or PO. IM administration causes necrosis.

O : By the IV route, delayed

D : The $t_{\frac{1}{2}}$ of digoxin is 40 hours (In anuric patients = 100 h)

CI : Contraindicated where heart block already exists

C : Atrio-ventricular block, bradycardia

S : N and V, confusion, visual deflects

E : Renal

I : Hypokalaemia enhances the effect of digoxin, so beware the effect of concurrently-administered diuretics; binding competes with amiodarone, verapamil, nifedipine; absorption competes with antacids

GU: Safe; doesn't cross placenta or into milk

•••••••••••••••••••••••••••••

REMIFENTANIL

P : Not yet available

C : 4-anilidopiperidine (cf. fentanyl)

A : Pure µ agonist.

U : Interoperative analgesia and for analgesia in highly monitored areas

D : 0.025 - 0.05 µg/kg/min

R : IV (as glycine is used as a preservative at present it will not be suitable for spinal use in this formulation)

O : Rapid

D : Ultra short ($t_{\frac{1}{2}}\beta$ 10-20min), and importantly its duration of action does not increase with prolonged use (i.e. its context-sensitive half-life is constant, unlike either fentanyl or alfentanil)

C : As all opiates, but with a high incidence of skeletal rigidity with bolus doses of 2 µg/kg or greater

E : It is broken-down rapidly by cholinesterase to form metabolites with 1/300 to 1/1000th the potency. It is not a substrate of butyrylcholinesterase (pseudo-cholinesterase) and so its clearance should not be affected by cholinesterase deficiency or the administration of anti-cholinesterases

•••••••••••••••••••••••••••••

DESFLURANE

P : Clear colourless liquid with no preservatives. A boiling point of 23.5°C means that it requires a specially designed vaporiser

C : $CF_3-CFH-O-CHF_2$

U : Inhalational anaesthesia

D : MAC of 7%, reduced to 3.5% by 60% N_2O

R : Inhalation

O : As the blood:gas solubility of the drug is very low (0.42) desflurane would be expected to have a very fast onset of action and therefore be ideal for inhalational induction of anaesthesia, however the high incidence of coughing, breath-holding, laryngospasm and salivation reduce the ability to 'overpressure' so inhalational induction is no faster that halothane.

CI : As for other inhalational agents. Its use in neurosurgery is under review

C : No evidence of tissue toxicity (cf. halothane hepatitis). CVS effects are similar to isoflurane except for a marked increase in sympathetic activity (with tachycardia, hypertension and possibly raised intracranial pressure) on rapidly increasing the dose from 1 to 1.5 MAC. Respiratory effects are similar to isoflurane except for the increased irritation noted above. At 1 MAC desflurane does raise the intracranial pressure in some neurosurgical patients so is use in this field is questioned.

E : Is quicker than other volatile anaesthetic agents due to the poor tissue solubilities, so allowing particularly fast recovery even after prolonged anaesthesia. Metabolism is almost non-existent (0.004%)

I : Nil

GU: As other volatile agents desflurane causes uterine relaxation in a dose-dependant manner

•••••••••••••••••••••••••••••••

TRAMADOL

C : Aminocyclohexanol derivative

A : Moderate μ agonist, with weak κ and σ action Strong monoamine re-uptake activity; these two actions may relate to the two stereoisomers

U : Mild to moderate pain

R : Oral, rectal, IV, subcutaneous, IM, epidural

O : (Oral) peak action at 1h

D : (Oral) 4h

C : Less respiratory depression, constipation or sedation than other opiates; little or no analgesic tolerance and low potential for abuse

•••••••••••••••••••••••••••••••

SEVOFLURANE

P : Clear colourless liquid. Only recently licenced in the UK but in regular use in Japan where it has been licensed since 1990.

C : $(CF_3)2CH-O-CH_2F$

A : As other volatile anaesthetic agents

U : Inhalational anaesthesia

D : MAC 2%

R : Inhalation

O : As the blood:gas solubility of the drug is very low (0.6), and sevoflurane is not pungent or irritant like desflurane, it is the ideal agent for rapid trouble-free inhalational induction of anaesthesia.

CI : As for other inhalational agents. Its use with soda-lime is controversial as it reacts with alkali soda-lime at high temperature to form products found to be toxic to the lungs and kidneys of rats. The toxicity has not been shown in humans, and sevoflurane is probably less toxic with soda-lime than halothane which has been use for many years without problem

C : CVS and RS effects similar to isoflurane

E : It is metabolised in the liver (2%) and may exhibit hepatotoxicity, though no cases have been reported yet. Free flouride ions are also produced by sevoflurane metabolism, so there is a theoretical risk of nephrotoxicity, but the concentrations released are lower than enflurane

I : Nil

GU: As other volatile agents sevoflurane causes uterine relaxation in a dose-dependant manner

••••••••••••••••••••••••••••••

ROCURONIUM

P : As yet unlicensed

C : Steroidal relative of vecuronium

U : Neuromuscular blockade especially when rapid onset is a benefit

D : 0.6-0.9mg/kg

R : IV

O : Rapid (reliable intubating conditions in 60-90 sec with 0.6mg/kg)

D : Intermediate (27-53min)

CI : As other non-depolarising neuromuscular blocking agents, pregnancy

C : Few - no histamine release and haemodynamically stable

Although it may rival suxamethonium for rapid sequence induction it does not have a short duration of action and so should not be used in cases where rapid return of neuromuscular function may be required.

••••••••••••••••••••••••••••

MIVACURIUM

P : Clear colourless liquid, 2mg/ml

C : Ester analogue of atracurium

A : A non-depolarising neuromuscular blocking agent

U : Muscle relaxation for short procedures, and for intubation where spontaneous ventilation is desirable

D : 0.2-0.25 mg/kg for intubation, and 4.7-8.3 mg/kg/min for infusion, although the use of a nerve stimulator is recommended as there is a wide range of response

R : IV

O : 2-3 min (similar to atracurium)

D : Approx. twice as long as suxamethonium and half as long as atracurium - 21min to 25% recovery. No cumulation with repeated dosing. The duration is reduced to approximately 10min with neostigmine

CI : As other non-depolarising muscle relaxants, also anyone with a history of prolonged block after suxamethonium

C : Histamine release (similar to atracurium) leading to hypotension. Prolonged block in plasma cholinesterase deficiency or conditions associated with reduction in cholinesterase activity (liver and renal failure, pregnancy, CCF, carcinoma, burns, etc)

E : Ester hydrolysis by plasma cholinesterase

I : Those drugs that inhibit plasma cholinesterase including anticholinesterase, cytotoxics, ester-type local anaesthetics, oral contraceptive pill

....

ONDANSETRON

P : Clear colourless, 2mg/ml

A : 5-HT3 receptor antagonist whose action may be peripherally in the GI tract

U : Chemotherapy-induced emesis, post-operative nausea and vomiting

D : 4-8mg bolus

R : IV or PO

D : Medium ($t_{\frac{1}{2}}\beta$ 3h)

C : Nil

....

INDEX